VEGETARIAN DIET FOR WOMEN

COMPREHENSIVE GUIDE TO FOLLOWING A VEGETARIAN DIET WITH SPECIFIC RECIPES DESIGNED FOR WOMEN'S METABOLISM, IMPROVE HEALTH AND LOSE WEIGHT

By

Jim MOON

TABLE OF CONTENS

VEGETARIAN DIET GUIDE
HEALTH BENEFITS OF VEGETARIAN DIET

I've already mentioned some of the health benefits but let me back it up with some science. Of course, as mentioned earlier, if you eat only processed foods packed with sugar and saturated and trans-fat, eat little to no vegetables and fruits, and don't meet your macronutrient targets, you won't reap the benefits.

Boosts Heart Health

Following a plant-based diet makes you up to one-third less likely to end up in the hospital or die due to heart disease (Crowe et al., 2013). It all comes down to eating foods that will keep your blood sugar levels stable. High-fiber whole grains, nuts, legumes, and low-glycemic foods, in general, will reduce your overall risk of heart disease and lower your cholesterol (Harvard Medical School, 2020).

Reduces Cancer Risk

Vegetarians may have the upper hand when it comes to fighting off cancer (Tantamango-Bartley et al., 2013). This study found that plant-based diets don't only reduce your overall risk for cancer more than other diets; it is also more effective against female-specific cancers. Also, when it comes to Lacto- ovo vegetarians, they have a smaller chance of getting cancers of the gastrointestinal tract.

The consensus is that a diet filled with fresh fruits and veggies is key to combating cancer, and, of course, being a vegetarian makes it easier for you to get the recommended five servings a day.

Although the benefit isn't that significant, it is worth mentioning since every bit helps in the fight against the "big C."

Prevents Type 2 Diabetes

Following a healthy plant-based diet may prevent type 2 diabetes (Chiu et al., 2018). In fact, you have half the risk of developing this disease (Tonstad et al., 2013), and the good news doesn't stop there. If you already suffer from this disease, a vegetarian diet will help treat the associated symptoms and may even reverse the disease entirely (Jenkins et al., 2003).

Eating foods that keep your blood sugar levels steady is the secret behind preventing type 2 diabetes—something you'll be doing a lot of when you follow a vegetarian diet.

Lowers Blood Pressure

Plant foods are lower in fat and contain less sodium and cholesterol, which means they will help lower your blood pressure. Furthermore, fruits and veggies contain high potassium concentrations, which also help to lower blood pressure. Studies show that following a plant-based diet, primarily vegan, leads to lower blood pressure than those who consume animal products (Appleby et al., 2002).

Helps with Asthma

Animal foods trigger an allergy or inflammatory response in the body, so removing these foods from your diet will have a positive impact overall. One study (albeit an older one) found 22 out of 24 participants were less dependent on their asthma medication after adopting the vegetarian lifestyle (Lindahl et al., 1985).

Improves Your Mood

A lot of factors come into play when it comes to your mood—what you eat, how active you are, as well as your sleeping pattern. Since animal products are chemical-laden, cutting them from your diet will have a mood-boosting effect.

Increases Energy Levels Elevated energy levels are one of the most celebrated changes I noticed after switching to a vegetarian diet. There aren't enough hours in the day, but when you follow a plant-based diet, you have enough energy to do everything, and then some. Fruits and vegetables are high in vitamins and antioxidants, and this will give you a significant energy boost. The fact that your digestion will also run better due to the increased fiber will add to your newly-found get-up-and-go attitude!

Supports Better Sleep

Meat is heavy and can slow down digestion. When your body doesn't need to digest such dense proteins, you'll enjoy a better night's sleep. The speedier breakdown of plant protein also means your body will get all the minerals it needs for some much-needed shuteye. Add to that the fact that most vegetarians generally lead a healthier lifestyle—drink less, don't smoke, exercise regularly, etc., and counting sheep will be a thing of the past.

Improve Bone Health Osteoporosis is a leading cause of bone weakness, and this is caused by the removal of calcium from the bone and eventually leading to a hole in the bone. This condition is greatly reduced in people with a vegetarian diet. Eating animal products can lead to osteoporosis by forcing calcium out of the bone and eventually leading to less bone mineral. Those are some pretty amazing health benefits, right? And they're not the only ones—more and more studies are coming out documenting the positive bodily changes you'll experience if you cut out meat. Even a little goes a long way if you don't want to go full-blown vegetarian, try to steer your diet in a direction where the focus is more on fruits and veggies and less on meat. The Mediterranean diet comes to mind here!

WHAT TO EAT: MACRO- AND MICRO-NUTRIENTS

Since the standard American diet is built around animal protein, it's hard for most people to understand how vegetarians who reduce the ingredients they consider essential to a healthy diet will get the nutrients their bodies need. In fact, saturated fat and trans-fat in animal protein, antibiotics, chemicals, cholesterol, etc. are all harmful to the human body. If you learn about this, you will have to change your thinking about eating again In order to scientifically adjust your eating habits, I hope you have an understanding of protein, carbohydrates and fats, and understand how each nutrient is essential to the function of the body.

The best macronutrient breakdown for a vegetarian diet is as follows:

25% protein

45% carbohydrates

30% fat

If you're not sure what this means, you will need to work out how many calories your body needs per day to function at an optimal level. This depends on your body shape, age, activity level, etc. There are various calorie counters online that will help you calculate your daily caloric needs. Once you have this number, you just divide it in the above percentages, and "Bob's your uncle," as they say!

You will find people who will tell you that the vegetarian diet is too high in carbs. Well, not all carbs are the same Let me break down the various macronutrients and how much you need to eat to stay healthy. Afterward, we will look closer at the micronutrients.

Protein

Many vegetarians, both new and old, always have to deal with the problem of getting enough protein in their diet. The most important part of this is the confusion of how to deal with the choice of protein.

We both understand that protein is an essential part of a person's balanced diet. And most of our protein as humans comes from animals. But where will you get your protein from if you can't rely on a thick slice of steak? The truth is there are good numbers of protein sources from plants. As vegetarians, we have access to a wider variety of proteins, such as:

Tofu is the most familiar source of non-meat protein for a lot of vegetarians but believe me; there are many others I have tried and which you can too. Cooked Lentils; Cooked Beans; Whole Grain Pasta; Nuts; Eggplant; Tofu; Ground Flaxseed; Mushroom; Cauliflower; and Cooked Quinoa are some of the best sources of plant protein that you can add to maintain a balanced meal

It should now be clear that the belief that plant-based protein won't be enough to sustain your body's protein needs is unfounded. Ultimately, the building blocks of both types of protein (amino acids) are the same—on a cellular level, your body won't be able to tell the difference. Furthermore, when your body breaks down the amino acids in the food, it will build complete proteins. This also smashes the myth that you'll need to eat various proteins in one sitting to 'mimic' animal protein.

Carbohydrates

As I mentioned before, not all carbohydrates are created equal. Our body needs carbohydrates to function properly, but you must choose the right type of carbohydrates to get the best results. When choosing carbohydrates, the more natural the ingredients, the better for the body, because the simplicity of processing and packaging contains almost no fiber. However, foods rich in plant fiber, vitamins, minerals and phytonutrients can help your body resist oxidation and inflammation. Fiber content can slow down the digestion of carbohydrates and control the rise of blood sugar in the body. Eating high- fiber carbohydrates regularly helps you prevent type 2 diabetes, fight cancer, and keep your body in good condition.

As you read above, 45 percent of your daily calories should go to carbohydrates. If you follow a 2,000-calorie diet, you'll be eating 225 grams of carbs a day. However, you may end up eating more on a vegetarian diet, then you need to keep an eye on your carb intake to prevent weight gain.

Fat

I know you've been told that fat makes fat and leads to high cholesterol actually, people have misunderstood the role of fat for a long time. What's more, fat plays a vital role in your health. Fat is essential for the absorption of fat-soluble vitamins, cell growth, hormone production, and digestion. Research showed that eating good fats (polyunsaturated and monounsaturated) can help lose weight, reduce inflammation, fight depression and anxiety, and improve your overall health (Manikam, 2008).

Now that you know the importance of fat, I will tell you how to meet your daily fat needs from a vegetarian diet. First of all, it needs to be clear where we get good fats? Some foods include avocado (20 grams per 100 grams), soybeans (3.3 grams per cup), olives (3.2 grams per 28 grams) and pumpkin seeds (14 grams per tablespoon), both are good sources of fat. Another important thing is how to control the intake of fat in daily cooking.

☐Sauté food using water or vegetable broth. Make sure to check the liquid level frequently you don't want your food to burn. Just keep adding water or broth until your food is cooked. Fruit or vegetable purée and applesauce are great oil substitutes when you're baking. It will keep your cakes and other baked goods moist.

☐If you're grilling something in the oven, I highly recommend getting a silicone mat to line your pan with. You can also use parchment paper to create the perfect non-stick environment for your oil-free grilling.

☐Invest in some non-stick cookware to help make cooking without oil less problematic. Okay, that covers your daily macronutrients. I think it's time we look at the vitamins and minerals (micronutrients) your body needs.

☐Vitamins and Minerals

As I mentioned before and will highlight throughout this cookbook, you need to focus on eating a wide variety of whole grains, fruits, vegetables, and fats with a particular focus on meeting your protein target if you want to get in all the nutrients your body needs. However, there are some nutrients you'll have to pay extra attention, or even consider supplementing.

Vitamin B-12

I want to take a moment to focus on vitamin B-12—a vital nutrient, which isn't found in many plant foods. If you decide to cut out all animal food sources, then you will have to consume more vitamin B-12-rich foods or you will have to supplement this vitamin. Since B-12 plays an important role in producing red blood cells and preventing anemia, I recommend you add a supplement to your diet just to be safe.

Omega-3 Fatty Acids

Before we move on to healthy foods you can't go wrong eating daily, let's look at omega-3s. To boost the health benefits of the vegetarian diet, getting in a good dose of fatty acids like docosahexaenoic acid (DHA), Eicosapentaenoic acid (EPA), and alpha-linolenic acid (ALA) is a must! Omega-3s help combat inflammation in the body, and through doing that, decrease your risk of getting heart disease or other issues caused by inflamed cells. When I first heard omega-3, I immediately thought about seafood, but I was pleasantly surprised that you could find ALA in various vegetarian sources.

HOW TO CHOOSE THE RIGHT FOOD FOR VEGETARIAN

Although all fruits and vegetables are superfoods as they're packed with nutrients our bodies love, some do stand out above the rest. Since making the healthiest choices is what you should aim for when following a vegetarian diet, you can boost your success rate by eating specific fruits and veggies daily, as well as focusing on herbs, spices, and drinks that have proven benefits.

I'll share with you some of the foods I attempt to eat daily and others I pack on my plate at least once a week.

Daily

Berries

Berries aren't only delicious, they're some of the healthiest foods on the planet. The number of health benefits packed in these juicy snacks is impressive. Not only do they contain essential nutrients, but they're also chock full of antioxidants that help keep free radicals at bay. What's a free radical, you ask? Well, they're rogue and unstable molecules that do you good in small numbers but will cause oxidative stress when their numbers get too high (LiveScience, 2016). This increases your risk of getting various diseases. But thanks to blueberries, blackberries, and raspberries and their high antioxidant content (the highest out of all common fruits), you can protect your cells (Wolfe et al., 2008).

Leafy greens

Kale, spinach, chard, and arugula are s78ome of the leafy-green superstars out there. They're low in calories but packed with vitamins, phytonutrients, and fiber. They're good for you in more ways than you can imagine. If the bulk of the veggies you eat is green and leafy, you can be sure to feel like a new person—even your skin will glow.

Nuts and seeds

Nuts and seeds are tiny yet powerful sources of protein, fat, fiber, vitamins, and minerals. What I appreciate most about these snacks is that I feel full and stay satiated for longer after eating only a handful. It's the perfect "tie-me- over" food when your tummy starts to grumble.

Turmeric

You've probably read about the wonders of turmeric or, more specifically, the active compound curcumin. This spice has scientifically been proven to have remarkable health benefits ranging from preventing heart disease, degenerative brain diseases, and can even help combat cancer cells. Its anti- inflammatory and antioxidant properties make it an anti-aging super spice.

Beans

If you ask me, one of the most underrated foods out there. Not only are beans and legumes high in dietary fiber, protein, vitamins, and minerals, they also contain B vitamins that you need as much of as you can get. Evidence suggests that beans' high fiber content will improve cholesterol levels and help your gut stay in good shape. Again, it comes down to managing those blood sugar levels!

Onions and garlic

You may not consider onions and garlic as nutritional powerhouses, but I am happy to convince you otherwise. Onions are high in potassium, folate, vitamin B6, and vitamin C. Garlic, on the other hand, contains all the goodies onions do with thiamin, calcium, phosphorus, copper, and manganese added to the mix!

And don't forget that it makes almost all savory dishes taste better.

Green tea

This wonder beverage is one of the healthiest on the planet. It comes loaded with antioxidants, which, as we've established, is terrific news for your overall health. Some of the health benefits of green tea include improved brain function, lowered risk of heart disease, protection against cancer, and better weight management (Chacko et al., 2010).

Once a Week

Ginger

Ginger is used in traditional and alternative medicine the world over, primarily when it comes to digestive health and fighting off nasty germs. Gingerol is the active compound in ginger and is responsible for all the medicinal properties. What makes it so powerful is the anti-inflammatory and antioxidant effects it has. You read about free radicals and oxidative stress and accompanied diseases earlier on, and now you have another food source to help heal your body!

Lemon juice

One of the main reasons why I can't do without lemon juice may surprise you. No, it's not for its vitamin C content but for its ability to combat anemia! Since vegetarians are prone to iron deficiency, including lemon juice in our diet will help with iron absorption from plant sources (Ballot et al., 1987). Your gut can absorb iron from animal protein, but it has a hard time doing so from plant-based sources. So, to help your body out a little, add lemon to your diet, as well as vitamin C and citric acid.

Dark chocolate

Who wouldn't want to eat chocolate once a week? I am not talking about overly sweet, processed, milk chocolate but the real deal—dark chocolate. The more unrefined the chocolate, the higher its flavanol content, and that's what we want. Flavanols are good for your arteries, and that makes them great for your heart and overall body. It tells your arteries to relax, and that reduces your blood pressure (Schewe et al., 2008). If you can recall, I suffered from hypertension when I first started following a vegetarian diet. Finding out that dark chocolate could help was delightful news!

Dates

This is another antioxidant-packed food, but that's not the only reason why I enjoy it once a week or so—dates make an excellent natural sweetener. Since they're dried, their sugar content is higher than fresh fruit, making them the perfect substitute for white sugar. Not to mention that they'll add some extra nutrients and fiber to any recipe you're preparing!

I usually make a date paste (recipe included in this cookbook) and substitute one cup of sugar with one cup of date paste.

However, you have to keep in mind that dried fruit overall has a much higher calorie content than their fresh counterparts. Furthermore, most of these calories come from carbs. That's my way of suggesting you don't overdo it when you eat this super sweet food—the vitamin, mineral, protein, and fiber content should blind you to the fact that it is a high-calorie food.

By now, you can understand my obsession too. I can be more serious once it comes to my vegetarian diet. In the pages that follow, there are mouth- watering recipes that will make you wonder why you didn't go meat-free ages ago. I also include some meal plans—something I found invaluable when I first started following the vegetarian diet. It makes it possible for you to stick to your guns and learn as you go along.

Note: This book has given you all the information you need to do this diet correctly and do it right. It is essential to understand what you are getting into when you embark on this diet, and this book gave you valuable information that you can use to your advantage and avoid the problems that can come with this diet. You want to stay healthy and make sure that your body can do what it needs to do. As with anything, we emphasize that if something seems wrong or unnatural, you will need to see a doctor to make sure you are safe and that your body can handle this diet. Use the knowledge in this book to get amazing recipes and learn directions for excellent meals for yourself. Consult your doctor before to starting new diet.

BREAKFAST RECIPES

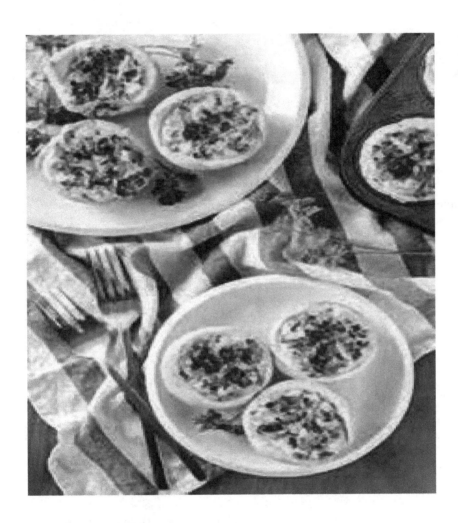

1) BREAKFAST SPINACH QUICHE

Preparation Time: 10 minutes   **Cooking Time:** 15 minutes   **Servings: 4**

Ingredients:
- ✓ 7 ounces whole wheat flour
- ✓ 7ounces spinach, torn
- ✓ 2.tablespoons olive oil
- ✓ 2tablespoons flax meal mixed with
- ✓ 3 tablespoons water

Directions:
- ❖ In your food processor, mix flour with half of the oil, flax meal, milk, salt and pepper and pulse well.
- ❖ Transfer to a bowl, knead a bit, cover and keep in the fridge for 10 minutes.
- ❖ Heat up a pan with the rest of the oil over medium-high heat
- ❖ Add onion, spinach, tofu, salt and pepper
- ❖ Stir, cook for a few minutes and take off heat.

Ingredients:
- ✓ 2 tablespoons almond milk
- ✓ 3 ounces soft tofu, crumbled
- ✓ Salt and black pepper to the taste
- ✓ 1 yellow onion, chopped

- ❖ Divide dough in 4 pieces, roll each piece
- ❖ Place on the bottom of a ramekin
- ❖ Divide spinach mix into the ramekins
- ❖ Place all ramekins in your Air Fryer's basket
- ❖ Cook at 360 °F for 15 minutes.
- ❖ Leave quiche aside to cool down a bit
- ❖ Then serve them for breakfast.

2) TOMATOES BREAKFAST SALAD

Preparation Time: 10 minutes   **Cooking Time:** 20 minutes   **Servings: 2**

Ingredients:
- ✓ 2 tomatoes, halved Cooking spray
- ✓ Salt and black pepper to the taste
- ✓ 1 teaspoon parsley, chopped
- ✓ 1 teaspoon basil, chopped

Directions:
- ❖ Spray tomato halves with cooking oil
- ❖ Season with salt and pepper
- ❖ Place them in your Air Fryer's basket
- ❖ Cook at 320 ° F for 20 minutes.

Ingredients:
- ✓ 1 teaspoon oregano, chopped
- ✓ 1 teaspoon rosemary, chopped
- ✓ 1 cucumber, chopped
- ✓ 1 green onion, chopped

- ❖ Transfer tomatoes to a bowl, add parsley, basil
- ❖ Then oregano, rosemary, cucumber and onion
- ❖ Toss and serve for breakfast.

3) BREAKFAST PIZZA

Preparation Time: 10 minutes   **Cooking Time:** 15 minutes   **Servings: 4**

Ingredients:
- ✓ 1 cup cauliflower, shredded
- ✓ 3 tablespoon almond flour
- ✓ ¼ teaspoon salt

Directions:
- ❖ Whisk the eggs and combine them together with almond flour, salt, and shredded cauliflower.
- ❖ Stir the mixture until smooth.
- ❖ Line the pizza mold with the baking paper and transfer the cauliflower dough inside it.
- ❖ Flatten the cauliflower crust gently.

Ingredients:
- ✓ 2 eggs, beaten
- ✓ 1 cup spinach, chopped
- ✓ 1 oz Parmesan

- ❖ Place the spinach over the pizza crust.
- ❖ Grate the cheese and sprinkle the spinach.
- ❖ Preheat the oven to 365F.
- ❖ Put the pizza in the oven and cook for 15 minutes or until cooked

4)   KETO PUMPKIN PANCAKES

Preparation Time: 10 minutes   **Cooking Time:** 6 minutes   **Servings: 8**

Ingredients:

- ✓ 2 tablespoons butter
- ✓ 1 teaspoon pumpkin spice
- ✓ 1 teaspoon baking powder
- ✓ 2 large eggs

Ingredients:

- ✓ ¼ cup sour cream
- ✓ 1 cup almond meal
- ✓ ¼ cup pumpkin puree
- ✓ 1/4 teaspoon salt

Directions:

- ❖ First in a mixing bowl combine your eggs, sour cream and butter
- ❖ In another mixing bowl, combine salt, almond meal, spice, baking powder
- ❖ Now slowly add your wet ingredients to your dry ingredients, while stirring to blend
- ❖ This will give you a sweet, smooth batter
- ❖ Over medium-heat warm up a cast-iron frying pan and grease it with butter
- ❖ Pour about 1/3 of your mixture into the skillet.

- ❖ When bubbles begin to form on top of the batter, allow it to
- ❖ Cook for about another minute, then flip it over
- ❖ Cook on the other side for an additional minute or so
- ❖ Repeat the previous last two steps until your batter is done
- ❖ Serve up your keto pumpkin pancakes with your favorite toppings.

5)   SCRAMBLED EGGS WITH CHEDDAR & SPINACH

Preparation Time: 8 minutes   **Cooking Time:** 10 minutes   **Servings: 1**

Ingredients:

- ✓ 1 tablespoon heavy cream
- ✓ 1 tablespoon olive oil
- ✓ 1 pinch of sea salt and pepper

Ingredients:

- ✓ 4 large eggs
- ✓ ½ cup cheddar cheese, shredded
- ✓ 4 cups spinach, chopped

Directions:

- ❖ Directions:
- ❖ Crack eggs into mixing bowl, along with heavy cream, salt, and pepper
- ❖ Mix. Heat a large pan over medium-high heat, adding olive oil
- ❖ When it is hot, add the spinach and let it sizzle and wilt adding some salt and pepper to it

- ❖ When the spinach is fully cooked, reduce heat to medium-low and add in the egg mixture
- ❖ Stir the eggs slowly and cook
- ❖ When the eggs have set, add in the cheese on top and allow it to melt.

6) WAFFLE/CINNAMON ROLL

Preparation Time: 5 minutes   **Cooking Time:** 6 minutes   **Servings: 1**

Ingredients:

Waffle:
- ✓ ½ teaspoon vanilla extract
- ✓ ½ teaspoon cinnamon
- ✓ ¼ teaspoon baking soda
- ✓ 2 large eggs
- ✓ 1 tablespoon erythritol
- ✓ 6 tablespoons almond flour

Directions:

- ❖ Add all the dry waffle Ingredients in a mixing bowl. In another mixing bowl, mix your wet Ingredients
- ❖ Ensure that they are combined well
- ❖ Then your wet Ingredients: to the dry Ingredients and blend well
- ❖ Heat your waffle iron. When waffle iron is hot, add your batter
- ❖ Remember to reserve 2 teaspoons of your waffle batter for the frosting

Ingredients:

Frosting:
- ✓ 2 teaspoons batter from waffles
- ✓ 2 tablespoons cream cheese
- ✓ 1 tablespoon heavy cream
- ✓ · ¼ teaspoon of cinnamon
- ✓ 1 tablespoon erythritol
- ✓ ¼ teaspoon vanilla extract

- ❖ While the waffle is cooking, add your cream cheese and erythritol to a small bowl
- ❖ Now add heavy cream, cinnamon, and batter
- ❖ 7Mix until smooth. Once the waffle is finished cooking, remove it from iron
- ❖ Place on serving the dish and spread frosting on top. Enjoy!

7) CREAMY ZUCCHINI NOODLES

Preparation Time: 10 minutes   **Cooking Time:** 5 minutes   **Servings: 4**

Ingredients:

- ✓ 3 medium zucchinis, use spiralizer to make noodles
- ✓ 1 tablespoon arrowroot powder
- ✓ ¼ teaspoon ground nutmeg
- ✓ Black pepper to taste

Directions:

- ❖ In a pan over medium-high heat melt butter
- ❖ Add in the garlic and cook for about 1 minute or until garlic softens
- ❖ Decrease the heat to medium- low.
- ❖ Then heavy cream, almond milk, nutmeg and stir well, bringing to a simmer
- ❖ In a mixing bowl, whisk 2 tablespoons of water and arrowroot powder until smooth
- ❖ Pour mixture into the pan and stir well

Ingredients:

- ✓ 1 teaspoon butter
- ✓ 2 garlic cloves, minced
- ✓ ½ cup almond milk, unsweetened
- ✓ ¾ cup parmesan cheese, grated

- ❖ Add black pepper and grated cheese and stir until cheese melts
- ❖ Pour sauce into a bowl, cover and set aside
- ❖ Heat pan over medium-high heat
- ❖ Once the pan is hot adding in zucchini noodles
- ❖ Stir until they soften, for about 5 minutes
- ❖ Now stir in the prepared sauce and serve.

8) FLAX CINNAMON MUFFINS

Preparation Time: 10 minutes   **Cooking Time:** 20 minutes   **Servings: 12**

Ingredients:

- ✓ 4 organic eggs, beaten
- ✓ 1/8 teaspoon salt
- ✓ 1 cup flax seed, ground
- ✓ ½ cup olive oil
- ✓ ½ cup coconut sugar
- ✓ ¼ cup coconut flour

Ingredients:

- ✓ 2 teaspoons vanilla
- ✓ 2 teaspoons cinnamon
- ✓ 1 teaspoon lemon juice
- ✓ ½ teaspoon baking soda
- ✓ 1 cup walnuts, chopped

Directions:

- ❖ Preheat your oven to 350°Fahrenheit
- ❖ Spray muffin pan with cooking spray and set aside
- ❖ Add all ingredients into a mixing bowl and mix well to combine

- ❖ Pour the batter into prepared muffin pan—filling each about full of mixture
- ❖ Bake for about 20 minutes. Serve and enjoy!

9) COCONUT WAFFLES

Preparation Time: 12 minutes   **Cooking Time:** 5 minutes   **Servings: 4**

Ingredients:

- ✓ 1/3 cup coconut flour
- ✓ ½ teaspoon salt
- ✓ 4 tablespoons butter, melted

Ingredients:

- ✓ 6 organic eggs
- ✓ 1/8 teaspoon Stevia drops
- ✓ ½ teaspoon baking powder

Directions:

- ❖ Add eggs along with butter into your blender and blend until well combined
- ❖ Pour egg mixture into mixing bowl
- ❖ Add coconut flour, Stevia, baking powder and salt

- ❖ Mix well. Set aside for 5 minutes.
- ❖ Heat your waffle iron, once it is hot pour batter
- ❖ Cook for 5 minutes or according to your waffle iron instructions
- ❖ Serve and enjoy!

10) BAKED CHEESY ARTICHOKES

Preparation Time: 10 minutes   **Cooking Time:** 45 minutes   **Servings: 6**

Ingredients:

- ✓ 1 cup spinach, chopped
- ✓ 1 cup almond milk
- ✓ 12 ounces canned artichokes, halved
- ✓ 2 garlic cloves, minced

Ingredients:

- ✓ ½ cup cashew cheese, shredded
- ✓ 1 tablespoon dill, chopped
- ✓ A pinch of salt and black pepper
- ✓ 2 teaspoons olive oil

Directions:

- ❖ Heat up a pan with the oil over medium heat
- ❖ Add the garlic, artichokes, salt and pepper, stir and cook for 5 minutes.
- ❖ Transfer this to a baking dish, add the spinach,

- ❖ Then almond milk and the other Ingredients
- ❖ Toss a bit, bake at 380 degrees F for 40 minutes
- ❖ Divide between plates and serve for breakfast.

11) EGGPLANT SPREAD

Preparation Time: 10 minutes   **Cooking Time:** 25 minutes   **Servings: 4**

Ingredients:

- ✓ 1 pound eggplants
- ✓ 2 tablespoons olive oil
- ✓ 4 spring onions, chopped

Ingredients:

- ✓ ½ teaspoon chili powder
- ✓ 1 tablespoon lime juice
- ✓ Salt and black pepper to the taste

Directions:

- ❖ Arrange the eggplants in a roasting pan
- ❖ Bake them at 400 degrees F for 25 minutes.
- ❖ Peel the eggplants, put them in a blender

- ❖ Add the rest of the ingredients
- ❖ Pulse well, divide into bowls and serve for breakfast.

12) EGGPLANT AND BROCCOLI CASSEROLE

Preparation Time: 10 minutes   **Cooking Time**: 35 minutes   **Servings: 4**

Ingredients:

- ✓ 1 pound eggplants, roughly cubed
- ✓ 1 cup broccoli florets
- ✓ 1 cup cashew cheese, shredded
- ✓ ¼ cup almond milk
- ✓ 2 scallions, chopped

Ingredients:

- ✓ 1 tablespoon olive oil
- ✓ 2 tablespoons flaxseed mixed with 2 tablespoons water
- ✓ 1 tablespoon cilantro, chopped
- ✓ Salt and black pepper to the taste

Directions:

- ❖ In a roasting pan, combine the eggplants with the broccoli
- ❖ Add the other ingredients except the cashew cheese and the almond milk and toss.
- ❖ In a bowl, combine the milk with the cashew cheese

- ❖ Stir, pour over the eggplant
- ❖ Mix, spread, introduce the pan in the oven
- ❖ Bake at 380 degrees F for 35 minutes.
- ❖ Cool the casserole down, slice and serve.

13) CREAMY AVOCADO AND NUTS BOWLS

Preparation Time: 5 minutes   **Cooking Time**: 0 minutes   **Servings: 4**

Ingredients:

- ✓ 1 tablespoon walnuts, chopped
- ✓ 1 tablespoon pine nuts, toasted
- ✓ 2 avocados, peeled, pitted and roughly cubed
- ✓ 1 tablespoon lime juice

Ingredients:

- ✓ 1 tablespoon avocado oil
- ✓ Salt and black pepper to the taste
- ✓ ¼ cup coconut cream

Directions:

- ❖ In a bowl, combine the avocados with the nuts and the other ingredients

- ❖ Toss, divide into smaller bowls and serve for breakfast.

14) AVOCADO AND WATERMELON SALAD

Preparation Time: 5 minutes   **Cooking Time**: 0 minutes   **Servings: 4**

Ingredients:

- ✓ 2 cups watermelon, peeled and roughly cubed
- ✓ 2 avocados, peeled, pitted and roughly cubed
- ✓ 1 tablespoon lime juice

Ingredients:

- ✓ 1 tablespoon avocado oil
- ✓ ¼ cup almonds, chopped

Directions:

- ❖ In a bowl, combine the watermelon with the avocados and the other ingredients

- ❖ Toss and serve for breakfast.

15) CHIA AND COCONUT PUDDING

Preparation Time: 10 minutes   **Cooking Time**: 0 minutes   **Servings: 4**

Ingredients:

- ✓ ¼ cup walnuts, chopped
- ✓ 2 cups coconut milk
- ✓ ¼ cup coconut flakes

Ingredients:

- ✓ 3 tablespoons chia seeds
- ✓ 1 tablespoon stevia
- ✓ 1 teaspoon almond extract
- ❖ Toss, leave aside for 10 minutes and serve for breakfast.

Directions:

- ❖ In a bowl, combine the milk with the coconut flakes and the other ingredients

16) TOMATO AND CUCUMBER SALAD

Preparation Time: 5 minutes   **Cooking Time:** 0 minutes   **Servings: 4**

Ingredients:

- ✓ 2 cups cherry tomatoes, halved
- ✓ 2 cucumbers, sliced
- ✓ 1 tablespoon lime juice
- ✓ A pinch of salt and black pepper

Directions:

- ❖ In a bowl, combine the tomatoes with the cucumbers and the other ingredients

Ingredients:

- ✓ 1 tablespoon olive oil
- ✓ ½ cup kalamata olives, pitted and halved
- ✓ 1 tablespoon chives, chopped

- ❖ Toss, and serve for breakfast.

17) WALNUTS AND OLIVES BOWLS

Preparation Time: 5 minutes   **Cooking Time:** 0 minutes   **Servings: 4**

Ingredients:

- ✓ 1 cup walnuts, roughly chopped
- ✓ 1 cup black olives, pitted and halved
- ✓ 1 cup green olives, pitted and halved
- ✓ 1 tablespoon lime juice
- ✓ 1 teaspoon chili powder

Directions:

- ❖ In a bowl, mix olives with the walnuts and the other ingredients

Ingredients:

- ✓ 1 teaspoon rosemary, dried
- ✓ 1 teaspoon cumin, ground
- ✓ 2 spring onions, chopped
- ✓ 1 tablespoon cilantro, chopped
- ✓ A pinch of salt and black pepper
- ✓ 2 tablespoons avocado oil

- ❖ Toss, divide into smaller bowls and serve for breakfast.

18) KALE AND BROCCOLI PAN

Preparation Time: 5 minutes   **Cooking Time:** 12 minutes   **Servings: 4**

Ingredients:

- ✓ 1 cup broccoli florets
- ✓ 2 shallots, chopped
- ✓ 1 tablespoon olive oil
- ✓ 1 teaspoon sweet paprika
- ✓ 1 teaspoon turmeric powder

Directions:

- ❖ Heat up a pan with the oil over medium heat
- ❖ Add the shallots and sauté for 2 minutes.

Ingredients:

- ✓ 1 cup kale, torn
- ✓ Salt and black pepper to the taste
- ✓ ¼ cup cashew cheese, grated
- ✓ 2 tablespoons chives, chopped

- ❖ Then the broccoli, kale and the other ingredients, toss
- ❖ Cook for 10 minutes more, divide between plates and serve.

19) SPINACH AND BERRIES SALAD

Preparation Time: 5 minutes   **Cooking Time:** 0 minutes   **Servings: 4**

Ingredients:

- ✓ 1 cup baby spinach
- ✓ 1 cup blackberries
- ✓ 1 cup blueberries
- ✓ 1 tablespoon avocado oil

Directions:

- ❖ In a salad bowl, combine the spinach with the berries and the other ingredients

Ingredients:

- ✓ 1 tablespoon balsamic vinegar
- ✓ 1 tablespoon parsley, chopped
- ✓ ½ cup pine nuts, chopped
- ✓ Salt and black pepper to the taste
- ❖ Toss and serve for breakfast.

20) CAULIFLOWER HASH

Preparation Time: 10 minutes **Cooking Time:** 15 minutes **Servings: 4**

Ingredients:

- ✓ 2 cups cauliflower florets, roughly chopped
- ✓ ½ teaspoon basil, dried
- ✓ 1 teaspoon sage, dried
- ✓ 2 spring onions, chopped
- ✓ 1 tablespoon avocado oil

Directions:

- ❖ Heat up a pan with the oil over medium heat,
- ❖ Add the onions and sauté for 5 minutes.
- ❖ Then the cauliflower and the other ingredients, toss

Ingredients:

- ✓ ½ cup coconut cream
- ✓ ½ teaspoon sweet paprika
- ✓ Salt and black pepper to the taste
- ✓ 1 tablespoon cilantro, chopped

- ❖ Cook everything for 10 minutes more
- ❖ Divide between plates and serve for breakfast.

LUNCH RECIPES

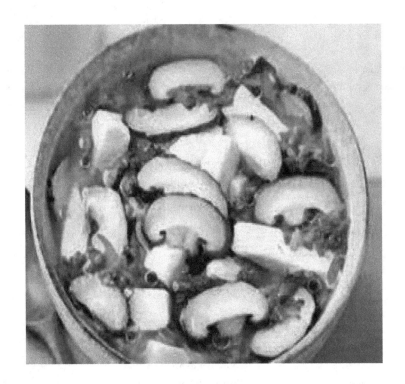

21) TOMATO AND PEPPERS PANCAKES

Preparation Time: 10 minutes   **Cooking Time:** 10 minutes   **Servings: 4**

Ingredients:

- ✓ 3 scallions, chopped
- ✓ 1 pound tomatoes, crushed
- ✓ 1 red bell pepper, chopped
- ✓ 1 green bell pepper, chopped
- ✓ Salt and black pepper to the taste

Directions:

- ❖ In a bowl, combine the tomatoes with the peppers
- ❖ Add the other ingredients except 1 tablespoon oil and stir really well.
- ❖ Heat up a pan with the remaining oil over medium heat, then ¼ of the batter

Ingredients:

- ✓ 1 teaspoon coriander, ground
- ✓ 2 tablespoons almond flour
- ✓ 2 tablespoons flaxseed mixed with
- ✓ 3 tablespoons water
- ✓ 3 tablespoons coconut oil, melted
- ❖ Spread into the pan
- ❖ Cook for 3 minutes on each side and transfer to a plate.
- ❖ Repeat this with the rest of the batter
- ❖ Transfer all pancakes to a platter and serve.

22) GREENS AND VINAIGRETTE

Preparation Time: 10 minutes   **Cooking Time:** 0 minutes   **Servings: 4**

Ingredients:

- ✓ 1 cup baby kale
- ✓ 1 cup baby arugula
- ✓ 1 cup romaine lettuce
- ✓ 2 tomatoes, cubed
- ✓ 1 cucumber, cubed

Directions:

- ❖ In a bowl, combine the oil with the vinegar, lime juice
- ❖ Then salt and pepper and whisk well.

Ingredients:

- ✓ 3 tablespoons lime juice
- ✓ 1/3 cup olive oil
- ✓ 1 tablespoon balsamic vinegar
- ✓ Salt and black pepper to the taste
- ❖ In another bowl, combine the greens with the vinaigrette
- ❖ Toss and serve right away.

23) MUSHROOM AND MUSTARD GREENS MIX

Preparation Time: 10 minutes   **Cooking Time:** 20 minutes   **Servings: 4**

Ingredients:

- ✓ 1 pound white mushrooms, halved
- ✓ 2 cups mustard greens
- ✓ 1 tablespoon lime juice
- ✓ 3 scallions, chopped
- ✓ 2 tablespoons olive oil

Directions:

- ❖ Heat up a pan with the oil over medium heat
- ❖ Add the scallions, paprika, garlic and parsley and sauté for 5 minutes.

Ingredients:

- ✓ 1 teaspoon sweet paprika
- ✓ 1 teaspoon rosemary dried
- ✓ 2 bunches parsley, chopped
- ✓ 3 garlic cloves, minced
- ✓ Salt and black pepper to the taste
- ❖ Then the mushrooms and the other Ingredients, toss
- ❖ Cook over medium heat for 15 minutes, divide between plates and serve.

24) CHARD AND GARLIC SAUCE

Preparation Time: 10 minutes   **Cooking Time**: 15 minutes   **Servings: 4**

Ingredients:

- ✓ ½ cup walnuts, chopped
- ✓ 4 cups red chard, torn
- ✓ 3 tablespoons olive oil
- ✓ Juice of 1 lime
- ✓ 1 celery stalks, chopped

Directions:

- ❖ Heat up a pan with the oil over medium heat
- ❖ Add the scallions, garlic and the celery and sauté for 5 minutes.

Ingredients:

- ✓ 1 cup coconut cream
- ✓ 4 garlic cloves, minced
- ✓ 1 tablespoon balsamic vinegar
- ✓ 2/3 cup scallions, chopped
- ✓ A pinch of sea salt and black pepper
- ❖ Then the chard and the other Ingredients, toss
- ❖ Cook over medium heat for 10 minutes more
- ❖ Divide between plates and serve.

25) PARSLEY CHARD SALAD

Preparation Time: 10 minutes   **Cooking Time**: 0 minutes   **Servings: 4**

Ingredients:

- ✓ 1 pound red chard, steamed and torn
- ✓ 1 cup grapes, halved
- ✓ 1 cup cherry tomatoes, halved
- ✓ 1 celery stalk, chopped
- ✓ 3 tablespoons balsamic vinegar

Directions:

- ❖ In a bowl, combine the chard with the grapes, tomatoes

Ingredients:

- ✓ ½ cup coconut cream
- ✓ 1 teaspoon chili Powder
- ✓ 2 tablespoons olive oil
- ✓ ½ cup parsley, minced
- ✓ A pinch of sea salt and black pepper
- ❖ Add the other Ingredient
- ❖ Toss and serve right away.

26) BOK CHOY AND CAULIFLOWER RICE

Preparation Time: 10 minutes   **Cooking Time**: 20 minutes   **Servings: 4**

Ingredients:

- ✓ 2 tablespoons olive oil
- ✓ 2 garlic cloves, minced
- ✓ 4 scallions, chopped
- ✓ 2 cups cauliflower rice
- ✓ 1 cup bok choy, torn

Directions:

- ❖ Heat up a pan with the oil over medium heat
- ❖ Add the scallions and the garlic and sauté for 5 minutes.
- ❖ Then the cauliflower rice and the other Ingredients, toss

Ingredients:

- ✓ ½ cup cherry tomatoes, halved
- ✓ 2 tablespoons thyme, chopped
- ✓ 1 tablespoon lemon juice
- ✓ Zest of ½ lemon, grated
- ✓ A pinch of sea salt and black pepper
- ❖ Cook over medium heat for 15 minutes more
- ❖ Divide into bowls and serve.

27) HOT CRANBERRIES AND ARUGULA MIX

Preparation Time: 10 minutes   **Cooking Time**: 0 minutes   **Servings: 4**

Ingredients:

- ✓ 1 cup cranberries
- ✓ 2 cups baby arugula
- ✓ 1 avocado, peeled, pitted and cubed
- ✓ 1 cucumber, cubed

Directions:

- ❖ In a bowl, combine the arugula with the cranberries

Ingredients:

- ✓ ¼ cup kalamata olives, pitted and sliced
- ✓ 1 tablespoon walnuts, chopped
- ✓ 2 tablespoons olive oil
- ✓ 2 tablespoons lime juice
- ❖ Add the other Ingredients
- ❖ Toss well, divide between plates and serve.

28) CINNAMON CAULIFLOWER RICE, ZUCCHINIS AND SPINACH

Preparation Time: 10 minutes   **Cooking Time:** 10 minutes   **Servings: 4**

Ingredients:

- ✓ 1 cup cauliflower rice
- ✓ 2 tablespoons olive oil
- ✓ 1 zucchini, sliced
- ✓ 1 cup baby spinach
- ✓ ½ cup veggie stock
- ✓ ½ teaspoon turmeric powder

Ingredients:

- ✓ ¼ teaspoon cinnamon powder
- ✓ A pinch of sea salt and black pepper
- ✓ 1/3 cup dates, dried and chopped
- ✓ 1 tablespoon almonds, chopped
- ✓ ¼ cup chives, chopped

Directions:

- ❖ Heat up a pan with the oil over medium heat
- ❖ Add the cauliflower rice, dates, turmeric and cinnamon and sauté for 3 minutes.

- ❖ Then the zucchini and the other Ingredients, toss
- ❖ Cook the mix for 7 minutes more, divide between plates and serve.

29) ASPARAGUS, BOK CHOY AND RADISH MIX

Preparation Time: 10 minutes   **Cooking Time:** 12 minutes   **Servings: 4**

Ingredients:

- ✓ ½ pound asparagus, trimmed and halved
- ✓ 1 cup bok choy, torn
- ✓ 1 cup radishes, halved
- ✓ 2 tablespoons balsamic vinegar
- ✓ 2 tablespoons olive oil

Ingredients:

- ✓ 2 teaspoon Italian seasoning
- ✓ 2 teaspoons garlic powder
- ✓ 1 teaspoon coriander, ground
- ✓ 1 teaspoon fennel seeds, crushed
- ✓ 1 tablespoon chives, chopped

Directions:

- ❖ Heat up a pan with the oil over medium heat

- ❖ Add the asparagus, bok choy, the radishes and the other Ingredients, toss
- ❖ Cook for 12 minutes, divide between plates and serve.

30) KALE AND CUCUMBER SALAD

Preparation Time: 10 minutes   **Cooking Time:** 0 minutes   **Servings: 4**

Ingredients:

- ✓ 2 cups baby kale
- ✓ 2 cucumbers, sliced
- ✓ 2 tablespoons avocado oil

Ingredients:

- ✓ 1 cup coconut cream
- ✓ 1 teaspoon balsamic vinegar
- ✓ 2 tablespoons dill, chopped

Directions:

- ❖ In a bowl, combine the kale with the cucumbers

- ❖ Add the other Ingredients
- ❖ Toss and serve.

31) GARLIC MASHED POTATOES & TURNIPS

Preparation Time: 20 minutes   **Cooking Time:** 30 minutes   **Servings: 8**

Ingredients:

- ✓ 1 head garlic
- ✓ 1 teaspoon olive oil
- ✓ 1 lb. turnips, sliced into cubes
- ✓ 2 lb. potatoes, sliced into cubes
- ✓ ½ cup almond milk

Ingredients:

- ✓ ½ cup vegan parmesan cheese, grated
- ✓ 1 tablespoon fresh thyme, chopped
- ✓ 1 tablespoon fresh chives, chopped
- ✓ 2 tablespoons vegan butter
- ✓ Salt and pepper to taste

Directions:

- ❖ Preheat your oven to 375 degrees F.
- ❖ Slice the tip off the garlic head.
- ❖ Drizzle with a little oil and roast in the oven for 45 minutes.

- ❖ Boil the turnips and potatoes in a pot of water for 30 minutes or until tender
- ❖ Add all the ingredients to a food processor along with the garlic.
- ❖ Pulse until smooth.

32) GREEN BEANS WITH VEGAN BACON

Preparation Time: 15 minutes   **Cooking Time:** 20 minutes   **Servings: 8**

Ingredients:

- ✓ 2 slices of vegan bacon, chopped
- ✓ 1 shallot, chopped
- ✓ 24 oz. green beans
- ✓ Salt and pepper to taste

Ingredients:

- ✓ ½ teaspoon smoked paprika
- ✓ 1 teaspoon lemon juice
- ✓ 2 teaspoons vinegar

Directions:

- ❖ Preheat your oven to 450 degrees F.
- ❖ Add the bacon in the baking pan and roast for 5 minutes.
- ❖ Stir in the shallot and beans.
- ❖ Season with salt, pepper and paprika

- ❖ Roast for 10 minutes.
- ❖ Drizzle with the lemon juice and vinegar
- ❖ Roast for another 2 minutes.

33) COCONUT BRUSSELS SPROUTS

Preparation Time: 15 minutes   **Cooking Time:** 10 minutes   **Servings: 4**

Ingredients:

- ✓ 1 lb. Brussels sprouts, trimmed and sliced in half
- ✓ 2 tablespoons coconut oil

Ingredients:

- ✓ ¼ cup coconut water
- ✓ 1 tablespoon soy sauce

Directions:

- ❖ In a pan over medium heat, add the coconut oil
- ❖ Cook the Brussels sprouts for 4 minutes.

- ❖ Pour in the coconut water. Cook for 3 minutes.
- ❖ Add the soy sauce and cook for another 1 minute.

34) COD STEW WITH RICE & SWEET POTATOES

Preparation Time: 30 minutes   **Cooking Time:** 1 hour   **Servings: 4**

Ingredients:

- ✓ 2 cups water
- ✓ ¾ cup brown rice
- ✓ 1 tablespoon vegetable oil
- ✓ 1 tablespoon ginger, chopped
- ✓ 1 tablespoon garlic, chopped
- ✓ 1 sweet potato, sliced into cubes
- ✓ 1 bell pepper, sliced

Ingredients:

- ✓ 1 tablespoon curry powder
- ✓ Salt to taste
- ✓ 15 oz. coconut milk
- ✓ 4 cod fillets
- ✓ 2 teaspoons freshly squeezed lime juice
- ✓ 3 tablespoons cilantro, chopped

Directions:

- ❖ Place the water and rice in a saucepan.
- ❖ Bring to a boil and then simmer for 30 to 40 minutes. Set aside
- ❖ Pour the oil in a pan over medium heat.
- ❖ Cook the garlic for 30 seconds.
- ❖ Add the sweet potatoes and bell pepper

- ❖ Season with curry powder and salt. Mix well.
- ❖ Pour in the coconut milk. Simmer for 15 minutes.
- ❖ Nestle the fish into the sauce and cook for another 10 minutes
- ❖ Stir in the lime juice and cilantro.
- ❖ Serve with the rice.

35) VEGAN CHICKEN & RICE

Preparation Time: 15 minutes

Cooking Time: 3 hours and 30 minutes

Servings: 8

Ingredients:

- ✓ 8 Tofu thighs
- ✓ Salt and pepper to taste
- ✓ ½ teaspoon ground coriander
- ✓ 2 teaspoons ground cumin
- ✓ 17 oz. brown rice, cooked
- ✓ 30 oz. black beans

Ingredients:

- ✓ 1 tablespoon olive oil
- ✓ Pinch cayenne pepper
- ✓ 2 cups pico de gallo
- ✓ ¾ cup radish, sliced thinly
- ✓ 2 avocados, sliced

Directions:

- ❖ Season the tofu with salt, pepper, coriander and cumin
- ❖ Place in a slow cooker.
- ❖ Pour in the stock.
- ❖ Cook on low for 3 hours and 30 minutes

- ❖ Put the tofu in a cutting board. Shred the chicken.
- ❖ Toss the tofu shreds in the cooking liquid.
- ❖ Serve the rice in bowls, topped with the tofu and the rest of the ingredients.

36) RICE BOWL WITH EDAMAME

Preparation Time: 10 minutes

Cooking Time: 3 hours and 50 minutes

Servings: 6

Ingredients:

- ✓ 1 tablespoon coconut oil, melted
- ✓ ¾ cup brown rice (uncooked)
- ✓ 1 cup wild rice (uncooked)
- ✓ Cooking spray
- ✓ 4 cups vegetable stock
- ✓ 8 oz. shelled edamame

Ingredients:

- ✓ 1 onion, chopped
- ✓ Salt to taste
- ✓ ½ cup dried cherries, sliced
- ✓ ½ cup pecans, toasted and sliced
- ✓ 1 tablespoon red wine vinegar

Directions:

- ❖ Add the rice and coconut oil in a slow cooker sprayed with oil
- ❖ Pour in the stock and stir in the edamame and onions.
- ❖ Season with salt. Seal the pot.

- ❖ Cook on high for 3 hours and 30 minutes
- ❖ Stir in the dried cherries. Let sit for 5 minutes.
- ❖ Stir in the rest of the ingredients before serving.

37) CHICKPEA AVOCADO SANDWICH

Preparation Time: 10 minutes

Cooking Time: 5 minutes

Servings: 2

Ingredients:

- ✓ Chickpeas 1 can
- ✓ Avocado 1
- ✓ Dill, dried 25 teaspoon
- ✓ Onion powder 25 teaspoon
- ✓ Sea salt 5 teaspoon
- ✓ Celery, chopped 25 cup
- ✓ Green onion, chopped 25 cup

Ingredients:

- ✓ Lime juice 3 tablespoons
- ✓ Garlic powder 5 teaspoon
- ✓ Dark pepper, ground dash
- ✓ Tomato, sliced 1
- ✓ Lettuce 4 leaves
- ✓ Bread 4 slices

Directions:

- ❖ Drain the canned chickpeas and rinse them under cool water
- ❖ Place them in a bowl along with the herbs, spices, sea salt, avocado, and lime juice
- ❖ Use a potato masher or fork, mash the avocado and chickpeas together until you have a thick filling
- ❖ Try not to mash the chickpeas all the way, as they create texture.

- ❖ Stir the celery and green onion into the filling and prepare your sandwiches.
- ❖ Layout two slices of bread
- ❖ Top them with the chickpea filling, some lettuce, and sliced tomato.
- ❖ Top them off with the two remaining slices
- ❖ Slice the sandwiches in half, and serve.

38) ROASTED TOMATO SANDWICH

Preparation Time: 30 minutes   **Cooking Time:** 25 minutes   **Servings: 2**

Ingredients:

✓ Sourdough bread 4 slices
✓ Tomatoes, large, cut into eight rounds 2
✓ Avocado 1
✓ Sea salt 25 teaspoon
✓ Vegan mayonnaise 25 cup
✓ Garlic, minced 2 cloves

Directions:

❖ Begin by setting your electric cooker to Fahrenheit 350 degrees
❖ Lining an aluminum sheet pan with kitchen parchment
❖ Layout the sliced tomatoes on the sheet
❖ Sprinkle them with part of the salt, oregano
❖ Then pepper, and allow them to roast until tender, about fifteen minutes.
❖ Meanwhile, prepare the garlic aioli
❖ Whisk together the mayonnaise, garlic
❖ Add juice of lemon fruit, and some sea salt and pepper.
❖ Chill in the fridge until use.

Ingredients:

✓ Juice of lemon fruit 1 tablespoon
✓ Oregano, dried 25 teaspoon
✓ Black ground pepper 25 teaspoon
✓ Olive oil 2 tablespoons
✓ Fresh basil 25 cup
✓ Arugula 25 cup

❖ Use a pastry brush and coat one side of each slice of bread with the olive oil
❖ While doing this preheat a skillet over midway warmth
❖ Once hot, toast the bread oil-side down until browned
❖ Then remove them from the heat.
❖ To prepare the sandwiches, lay out the bread, oil side down
❖ On each slice spread the garlic aioli
❖ On half of the slices cover with the roasted tomatoes
❖ Add sliced avocado, basil, and arugula
❖ Top these slices with their matched slice without toppings
❖ Slice the sandwiches in half before serving.

39) QUINOA WITH CHICKPEAS AND TOMATOES

Preparation Time: 10 minutes   **Cooking Time:** 0 minute   **Servings: 6**

Ingredients:

✓ 1 tomato, chopped
✓ 1 cup quinoa, cooked
✓ ½ teaspoon minced garlic
✓ ¼ teaspoon ground black pepper
✓ ½ teaspoon salt

Directions:

❖ Take a large bowl, place all the ingredients in it, except for the parsley, and stir until mixed.

Ingredients:

✓ 1/2 teaspoon ground cumin
✓ 4 teaspoons olive oil
✓ 3 tablespoons lime juice
✓ 1/2 teaspoon chopped parsley

❖ Garnish with parsley and serve straight away.

40) BARLEY BAKE

Preparation Time: 10 minutes   **Cooking Time:** 98 minutes   **Servings: 6**

Ingredients:

✓ 1 cup pearl barley
✓ 1 medium white onion, peeled, diced
✓ 2 green onions, sliced
✓ 1/2 cup sliced mushrooms
✓ 1/8 teaspoon ground black pepper

Directions:

❖ Place a skillet pan over medium-high heat
❖ Add butter and when it melts, stir in onion and barley
❖ Then nuts and cook for 5 minutes until light brown.
❖ Join also mushrooms, green onions and parsley
❖ Sprinkle with salt and black pepper

Ingredients:

✓ 1/4 teaspoon salt
✓ 1/2 cup chopped parsley
✓ 1/2 cup pine nuts
✓ 1/4 cup vegan butter
✓ 29 ounces vegetable broth

❖ Cook for 1 minute and then transfer the mixture into a casserole dish.
❖ Pour in broth, stir until mixed
❖ Bake for 90 minutes until barley is tender and has absorbed all the liquid.
❖ Serve straight away

SNACK RECIPES

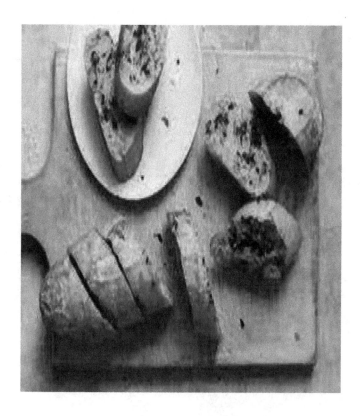

41) BLUEBERRY MUFFINS

Preparation Time: 10 minutes   **Cooking Time**: 35 minutes   **Servings: 12**

Ingredients:
- ✓ 1/2 cup unsweetened applesauce
- ✓ 1/4 cup soy margarine
- ✓ 1/2 tsp salt
- ✓ 2 cups flour

Directions:
- ❖ Preheat oven to 350 degrees Fahrenheit; line or grease 12 muffin cups.
- ❖ Combine margarine, applesauce, flour, salt, baking powder
- ❖ Then sugar, soy milk, and vanilla in a large mixing bowl

Ingredients:
- ✓ 1 cup sugar
- ✓ 1 tbsp baking powder
- ✓ 1/2 cup soy milk
- ✓ 1 tbsp vanilla extract
- ✓ 2 cups fresh blueberries

- ❖ Stir or blend well with an electric mixer.
- ❖ Fold in blueberries gently.
- ❖ Spoon into muffin cups until they are 3/4 of the way full
- ❖ Bake 35 minutes. Let cool 5 minutes. Serve.

42) BANANA MUFFINS

Preparation Time: 10 minutes   **Cooking Time**: 35 minutes   **Servings: 12**

Ingredients:
- ✓ 1 cup white sugar
- ✓ 1/2 cup brown sugar
- ✓ 3 cups flour
- ✓ 2 tsp baking powder
- ✓ 2 tsp ground cinnamon
- ✓ 1 tsp baking soda

Directions:
- ❖ Preheat oven to 350 degrees; grease or line 12 muffin cups.
- ❖ In a large bowl, stir together flour, both sugars, baking powder
- ❖ Then baking soda, cinnamon, nutmeg, and salt.

Ingredients:
- ✓ 1 tsp salt
- ✓ 1 tsp ground nutmeg
- ✓ 1 cup canola oil
- ✓ 2 cups mashed bananas
- ✓ 1 cup coconut milk

- ❖ In a separate bowl, combine canola oil, bananas, and coconut milk
- ❖ Stir banana mixture into flour mixture until just combined.
- ❖ Fill muffin cups with batter evenly. Bake for 35 minutes.
- ❖ Let cool for 5 minutes. Serve.

43) SAVORY VEGETABLE MUFFINS

Preparation Time: 10 minutes   **Cooking Time**: 20 minutes   **Servings: 24**

Ingredients:
- ✓ 1 cup flour
- ✓ 1 cup wheat flour
- ✓ 1/2 tsp salt
- ✓ 3/4 tsp baking soda
- ✓ 1/4 tsp cinnamon
- ✓ 1/4 tsp nutmeg
- ✓ 3/4 cup sugar
- ✓ 2 eggs

Directions:
- ❖ Preheat oven to 375 degrees Fahrenheit and grease or line 24 muffin cups
- ❖ Combine dry ingredients in a large bowl.
- ❖ Beat butter, sugar, vanilla, and eggs together in a mixer.
- ❖ Combine produce with applesauce and apple juice in a food processor and pulse until mixed.

Ingredients:
- ✓ 4 tbsp butter
- ✓ 1/8 cup apple juice
- ✓ 1 tsp vanilla extract
- ✓ 1 medium carrot
- ✓ 1/4 cup unsweetened applesauce
- ✓ 1/4 cup plain yogurt
- ✓ 2-1/2 cup vegetable puree

- ❖ Beat the carrots, puree, and yogurt into the butter mixture.
- ❖ Beat the dry ingredients into the wet ingredients until just combined.
- ❖ Scoop mixture into muffin tins. Bake for 20 minutes.
- ❖ Let cool 5 minutes. Serve.

44) PUFF PASTRY POCKETS

Preparation Time: 10 minutes   **Cooking Time:** 20 minutes   **Servings: 12**

Ingredients:
- ✓ 3 tbsp chopped green onions
- ✓ 8oz crumbled feta cheese
- ✓ 1 beaten egg

Ingredients:
- ✓ 17oz packaged frozen puff pastry, thawed
- ✓ 1 egg yolk, beaten with 1 tsp water

Directions:
- ❖ Preheat oven to 375 degrees Fahrenheit.
- ❖ Stir together feta with egg and green onions in a small bowl.
- ❖ Cut puff pastry into 12 squares and place a heaping tablespoon of feta mixture into the center of each one.

- ❖ Moisten pastry edges with water and fold over to form a triangle; press to seal with a fork.
- ❖ Brush pastries with egg yolk mixture. Bake for 20 minutes. Serve.

45) HUSH PUPPIES

Preparation Time: 10 minutes   **Cooking Time:** 35 minutes   **Servings: 12**

Ingredients:
- ✓ 1/2 cup white sugar
- ✓ 2 beaten eggs
- ✓ 1 diced onion

Ingredients:
- ✓ 1 cup self-rising cornmeal
- ✓ 1 cup self-rising flour
- ✓ 1 quart oil

Directions:
- ❖ Combine sugar with eggs and onion in a large bowl. Blend in cornmeal and flour.
- ❖ Heat 2 inches of oil to 365 degrees Fahrenheit in a skillet or pot on the stovetop.

- ❖ Drop batter in rounded teaspoons into hot oil.
- ❖ Fry until golden brown, then drain on paper towels. Serve warm.

46) CORN FRITTERS

Preparation Time: 10 minutes   **Cooking Time:** 40 minutes   **Servings: 12**

Ingredients:
- ✓ 1 cup sifted flour
- ✓ 3 cups vegetable oil
- ✓ 1 tsp baking powder
- ✓ 1/4 tsp white sugar

Ingredients:
- ✓ 1/2 tsp salt
- ✓ 1/2 cup milk
- ✓ 1 beaten egg
- ✓ 1 tbsp melted shortening
- ✓ 12oz canned whole kernel corn, drained
- ❖ Fold in corn kernels.

Directions:
- ❖ Heat oil in a pot or fryer to 365 degrees Fahrenheit.
- ❖ Combine flour in a large bowl with baking powder, sugar, and salt
- ❖ Beat in egg, shortening, and milk.

- ❖ Drop spoonfuls of batter into hot oil. Fry until golden, and drain.
- ❖ Serve warm.

47) GARLIC BREAD

Preparation Time: 10 minutes   **Cooking Time:** 10 minutes   **Servings: 10**

Ingredients:
- ✓ 1 pound Italian loaf bread
- ✓ 2 tsp olive oil
- ✓ 5 tbsp softened butter
- ✓ 3 crushed cloves of garlic
- ✓ 2 tsp olive oil

Ingredients:
- ✓ 1 cup shredded mozzarella
- ✓ 1 tsp dried oregano
- ✓ 1/4 tsp salt
- ✓ 1/4 tsp black pepper

Directions:
- ❖ Preheat oven broiler.
- ❖ Slice bread into thick slices, approximately ten per loaf.
- ❖ Combine olive oil with butter, oregano, garlic, salt, and pepper in a small bowl.

- ❖ Top each slice of bread evenly with the mixture.
- ❖ Arrange bread on a baking sheet and broil for 5 minutes until brown, being careful not to burn.
- ❖ Sprinkle over cheese and broil for 2 more minutes. Serve warm.

48) FRIED VEGGIE BREAD

Preparation Time: 10 minutes   **Cooking Time:** 15 minutes   **Servings: 4**

Ingredients:
- ✓ 1 chopped clove garlic
- ✓ 1/8 cup olive oil
- ✓ 1 cubed zucchini
- ✓ 1 cubed eggplant
- ✓ 1 chopped and seeded tomato

Ingredients:
- ✓ 2 tsp minced fresh oregano
- ✓ 1 tsp salt
- ✓ 2 tsp minced fresh basil
- ✓ 4 tsp garlic powder
- ✓ 6 tsp softened butter 1 French baguette

Directions:
- ❖ Cook garlic in olive oil in a large skillet over medium heat for 2 minutes
- ❖ Add zucchini and eggplant and fry for 5 more minutes.
- ❖ Then tomato, salt, basil, and oregano.
- ❖ Cook, stirring continuously, for 2 minutes, until tomato becomes pulpy. Preheat oven to 325 degrees Fahrenheit.

- ❖ Slice bread into 12 pieces and season evenly with garlic powder. Top evenly with butter.
- ❖ Heat bread in oven, directly on rack, for 3 minutes.
- ❖ Remove, top with vegetable mixture, and place on a serving platter.
- ❖ Serve warm.

49) SPINACH PUFFS

Preparation Time: 15 minutes   **Cooking Time:** 150 minutes   **Servings: 10**

Ingredients:
- ✓ 20oz frozen chopped spinach, thawed and drained
- ✓ 1 cup grated Parmesan
- ✓ 2 cups Italian bread crumbs
- ✓ 1/2 cup melted butter

Ingredients:
- ✓ 4 beaten eggs
- ✓ 4 chopped green onions
- ✓ 1/4 tsp salt
- ✓ 1/4 tsp black pepper

Directions:
- ❖ Preheat oven to 350 degrees Fahrenheit.
- ❖ Combine frozen chopped spinach with bread crumbs, butter, cheese, salt
- ❖ Then pepper, green onion, and eggs in a large bowl.

- ❖ Shape mixture into approximately 20 balls
- ❖ Place balls on a baking sheet.
- ❖ Bake for 15 minutes. Serve.

50) PARMESAN BREAD

Preparation Time: 10 minutes   **Cooking Time:** 15 minutes   **Servings: 8**

Ingredients:
- ✓ 1 tsp garlic salt
- ✓ 1/2 cup melted butter
- ✓ 1/4 tsp basil
- ✓ 1/4 tsp rosemary

Ingredients:
- ✓ 1/4 tsp garlic powder
- ✓ 1/4 tsp thyme
- ✓ 1 tbsp grated Parmesan
- ✓ 1 pound halved French bread loaf

Directions:
- ❖ Preheat oven to 350 degrees Fahrenheit.
- ❖ Combine garlic salt, butter, basil, rosemary, garlic powder, thyme, and Parmesan in a small bowl.
- ❖ Evenly sprinkle butter mixture over the bread halves. Top with additional Parmesan if desired.
- ❖ Place bread crust-down on baking sheet. Bake for 12 minutes. Serve.

51) SALTED ALMONDS

Preparation Time: 5 minutes   **Cooking Time:** 20 minutes   **Servings: 4**

Ingredients:
- ✓ 2 cups almonds
- ✓ 4 tablespoons salt

Ingredients:
- ✓ 1 cup boiling water

Directions:
- ❖ Stir the salt into the boiling water in a pan
- ❖ Add almonds in it and let them soak for 20 minutes.
- ❖ Then drain the almonds
- ❖ Spread them in an even layer on a baking sheet lined with baking paper and sprinkle with salt.
- ❖ Roast the almonds for 20 minutes at 300 degrees F
- ❖ Then cool them for 10 minutes and serve.

52) SPICED CHICKPEAS

Preparation Time: 45 Minutes   **Cooking Time:** 40 minutes   **Servings: 4**

Ingredients:
- ✓ Cayenne Pepper (.10 t.)
- ✓ Dried Oregano (.25 t.)
- ✓ Garlic Powder (.10 t.)

Ingredients:
- ✓ Salt (to Taste)
- ✓ Olive Oil (2 T.)
- ✓ Chickpeas (1 Can)

Directions:
- ❖ Start this recipe by prepping the oven to 450 and lining a baking sheet with parchment paper.
- ❖ Take a mixing bowl, add in chickpeas and coat with the spices and olive oil
- ❖ Once this is done, pop everything into the oven for 40 minutes.
- ❖ After 40 minutes, remove the pan from the oven, allow it to cool completely and enjoy.

53) LEMON & GINGER KALE CHIPS

Preparation Time: 30 Minutes   **Cooking Time:** 10 Minutes   **Servings: 5**

Ingredients:
- ✓ Ginger (1 t.)
- ✓ Salt (to Taste)
- ✓ Lemon Zest (1 t.)

Ingredients:
- ✓ Olive Oil (1 T.)
- ✓ Kale (7 Oz.)

Directions:

❖ Before you begin cooking this delicious snack, you'll want to prepare the oven to 300

❖ As this warms up, go ahead and line your baking sheet with parchment paper.

❖ Next, you are going to want to place your kale into a bowl

❖ Toss with the olive oil, lemon zest, ginger, and the salt

❖ Give everything a good toss to spread the seasonings over all of the kale.

❖ When the kale is set, spread it out evenly onto your baking sheet and pop into the oven for ten minutes

❖ By the end of this time, the edges of the leaves should look dry.

❖ If the kale is cooked to your liking, remove from the oven

❖ Allow to cool completely before serving.

54) CHOCOLATE ENERGY SNACK BAR

Preparation Time: 5 Minutes   **Cooking Time:** 0 Minutes   **Servings: 4**

Ingredients:
- ✓ Flax Seeds (1 T.)
- ✓ Chia Seeds (1 T.)
- ✓ Agave Nectar (2 T.)

Ingredients:
- ✓ Almonds (1 C.)
- ✓ Dried Cranberries (1 C.)
- ✓ Dates (1 C.)

Directions:

❖ When you need a snack that is easy to grab when you are on the go, this is the perfect recipe

❖ You are going to start out by pulsing the almonds and dates in a food processor

❖ Once they are chopped fine, add in the seeds, agave, and cranberries

❖ At this point, pulse until everything is combined.

❖ Next, you will want to add the batter into a lined pan

❖ Press everything down into the bottom.

❖ Finally, pop the dish into the fridge for two hours

❖ Cut into squares, and your bars are ready!

55) HAZELNUT & MAPLE CHIA CRUNCH

Preparation Time: 30 Minutes   **Cooking Time:** 5 Minutes   **Servings: 2**

Ingredients:
- ✓ Chia Seeds (.25 C.)
- ✓ Olive Oil (1 t.)
- ✓ Maple Syrup (.50 C.)

Ingredients:
- ✓ Hazelnuts (1.25 C.)
- ✓ Salt (to Taste)

Directions:

❖ To begin this recipe, start by heating a pan over medium heat

❖ Once warm, place the olive oil and maple in and bring to a boil.

❖ Once boiling, stir in your hazelnuts and cook on high for a minute or two

❖ After this time passes, add in the chia seeds and salt and cook for another three minutes.

❖ Now, turn the heat down to low

❖ Begin crushing the hazelnuts in the pan before pouring onto a lined cookie sheet

❖ At this point, try to spread the mixture evenly across the pan

❖ Then place it in the freezer for 15 minutes.

❖ Once the mixture has completely cooled, chop the ingredients into clusters and enjoy.

56) ROASTED CAULIFLOWER

Preparation Time: 30 Minutes   **Cooking Time:** 20 Minutes   **Servings: 4**

Ingredients:
- ✓ Olive Oil (1 T.)
- ✓ Cauliflower (1, Chopped)
- ✓ Salt (to Taste)

Ingredients:
- ✓ Smoked Paprika (2 t.)
- ✓ Parsley (2 T.)

Directions:

❖ If you like to snack, it is better to have healthier options at hand

❖ You'll want to start this recipe off by prepping your oven to 450.

❖ As this warms up, place the cauliflower florets into a large mixing bowl

❖ Toss with the olive oil, salt, and smoked paprika

❖ Once this is complete, lay it across a baking sheet and pop it into the oven for 20 minutes.

❖ When the cauliflower is cooked to your liking, remove from the oven

❖ Top with parsley, and you are all set.

57) APPLE CINNAMON CRISPS

Preparation Time: 2 Hours   **Cooking Time:** 2 Hours   **Servings: 2**

Ingredients:
- ✓ Cinnamon (1 t.)

Ingredients:
- ✓ Apple (1, Sliced)

Directions:

❖ This recipe is simple and delicious!

❖ You can start off by turning the oven to 200

❖ As this warms up, you'll want to prep a baking sheet with some parchment paper.

❖ With the baking sheet set, layout your apple slices across it evenly

❖ Sprinkle with the cinnamon

❖ Once this is done, pop the dish into the oven for two hours.

❖ Remove from oven, allow to cool, and enjoy.

58) PUMPKIN SPICE GRANOLA BITES

Preparation Time: 2 Hours   **Cooking Time:** 0 Minutes   **Servings: 4**

Ingredients:
- ✓ Pumpkin Pie Spice (.50 t.)
- ✓ Old-fashioned Rolled Oats (.75 C.)
- ✓ Medjool Dates (15)

Ingredients:
- ✓ Pumpkin Puree (.33 C.)
- ✓ Granola (.50 C.)

Directions:

❖ To start off, go ahead and place the oats into a food processor and process until it becomes flour

❖ Once this is done, you will want to add in the spice, pumpkin, and dates

❖ Puree everything again until you get a dough.

❖ From this dough, use your hands to take small bits and roll into ten balls

❖ Place the balls into the fridge for two hours and allow to firm up.

❖ Finally, roll the balls in your favorite granola and then enjoy

59) SALTED CARROT FRIES

Preparation Time: 30 Minutes   **Cooking Time:** 20 Minutes   **Servings: 4**

Ingredients:
- ✓ Olive Oil (2 T.)
- ✓ Salt (to taste)

Ingredients:
- ✓ Carrots (6)

Directions:
- ❖ Begin by prepping your oven to 425
- ❖ While this warms up, line a baking sheet with parchment paper and set to the side.
- ❖ Next, you will want to take your carrots and carefully cut them into smaller sections, resembling fries.
- ❖ Once the carrots are cut, you will want to toss them in a bowl with the salt and olive oil

- ❖ As you do this, make sure the carrots are evenly coated.
- ❖ Finally, pop the dish into the oven for twenty minutes
- ❖ By the end, the carrots should be slightly browned and cooked through
- ❖ If it is cooked to your liking, allow to cool and then enjoy.

60) ZESTY ORANGE MUFFINS

Preparation Time: 40 Minutes   **Cooking Time:** 20 Minutes   **Servings: 11**

Ingredients:
- ✓ Chopped Hazelnuts (3 T.)
- ✓ Orange Juice (1 C.)
- ✓ Olive Oil (.50 C.)
- ✓ Baking Powder (2 t.)
- ✓ Brown Sugar (.75 C.)

Ingredients:
- ✓ Flour (2 C.)
- ✓ Baking Soda (1 Pinch)
- ✓ Salt (to Taste)
- ✓ Orange Zest (2 T.)

Directions:
- ❖ Muffins are the perfect snack to grab and go when you need to leave the house quickly
- ❖ Start off by prepping the oven to 350.
- ❖ As this warms up, take out your mixing bowl
- ❖ Combine the hazelnuts, salt, baking soda, baking powder, sugar, and flour

- ❖ Once these are mixed together well, add in the olive oil and orange juice.
- ❖ With your mixture made, evenly pour into lined muffin tins
- ❖ Then pop it into the oven for 20 minutes.
- ❖ By the end, the muffins should be cooked through and golden at the top
- ❖ If they look done, remove from the oven, and your snack is ready to go.

DINNER RECIPES

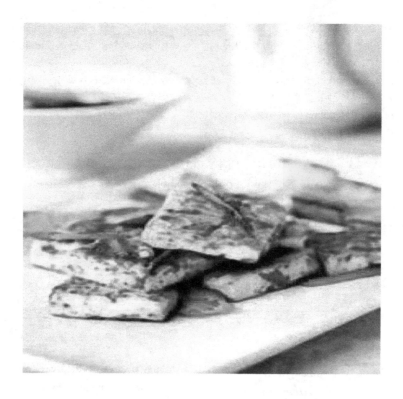

61) SPICY GRILLED TOFU STEAK

Preparation Time: 30 min   **Cooking Time**: 20 min.   **Servings: 4**

Ingredients:
- ✓ 1 tbsp. Of the following:
- ✓ Chopped scallion chopped cilantro soy sauce
- ✓ Hoisin sauce
- ✓ 2 tbsp. Oil
- ✓ ¼ t. Of the following:
- ✓ Salt

Ingredients:
- ✓ Garlic powder
- ✓ Red chili pepper powder
- ✓ Ground sichuan peppercorn powder
- ✓ ½ t. Cumin
- ✓ 1 pound firm tofu

Directions:
- ❖ Place the tofu on a plate and drain the excess liquid for about 10 minutes.
- ❖ Slice drained tofu into ¾ thick stakes.
- ❖ Stir the cumin, sichuan peppercorn, chili powder,
- ❖ Then garlic powder, and salt in a mixing bowl until well-incorporated.
- ❖ In another little bowl, combine soy sauce, hoisin, and 1 teaspoon of oil.
- ❖ Heat a skillet to medium temperature with oil

- ❖ Then carefully place the tofu in the skillet.
- ❖ Sprinkle the spices over the tofu, distributing equally across all steaks
- ❖ Cook for 3-5 minutes, flip, and put spice on the other side.
- ❖ Cook for an additional 3 Minutes.
- ❖ Brush with sauce and plate.
- ❖ Sprinkle some scallion and cilantro and enjoy.

62) PIQUILLO SALSA VERDE STEAK

Preparation Time: 30 min   **Cooking Time**: 25 min   **Servings: 8**

Ingredients:
- ✓ 4 ½ inch thick slices of ciabatta
- ✓ 18 oz. Firm tofu, drained
- ✓ 5 tbsp. Olive oil, extra virgin
- ✓ Pinch of cayenne
- ✓ ½ t. Cumin, ground
- ✓ 1 ½ tbsp. Sherry vinegar

Ingredients:
- ✓ 1 shallot, diced
- ✓ 8 piquillo peppers (can be from a jar) drained and cut to ½ inch strips
- ✓ 3 tbsp. Of the following:
- ✓ Parsley, finely chopped capers, drained and chopped

Directions:
- ❖ Place the tofu on a plate to drain the excess liquid, and then slice into 8 rectangle pieces.
- ❖ You can either prepare your grill or use a grill pan. If using a grill pan, preheat the grill pan.
- ❖ Mix 3 tablespoons of olive oil, cayenne, cumin, vinegar,
- ❖ Add shallot, parsley, capers, and piquillo peppers in a medium bowl to make our salsa verde
- ❖ Season to preference with salt and pepper.
- ❖ Use a paper towel, dry the tofu slices.

- ❖ Brush olive oil on each side, seasoning with salt and pepper lightly.
- ❖ Place the bread on the grill and toast for about 2 minutes using medium-high heat.
- ❖ Next, grill the tofu, cooking each side for about 3 minutes or until the tofu is heated through.
- ❖ Place the toasted bread on the plate then the tofu on top of the bread
- ❖ Gently spoon out the salsa verde over the tofu and serve.

63) BUTTERNUT SQUASH STEAK

Preparation Time: 30 min   **Cooking Time:** 50 min.   **Servings: 4**

Ingredients:
- ✓ 2 tbsp. Coconut yogurt
- ✓ ½ t. Sweet paprika
- ✓ 1 ¼ c. Low-sodium vegetable broth
- ✓ 1 sprig thyme
- ✓ 1 finely chopped garlic clove

Ingredients:
- ✓ 1 big thinly sliced shallot
- ✓ 1 tbsp. Margarine
- ✓ 2 tbsp. Olive oil, extra virgin
- ✓ Salt and pepper to liking

Directions:
- ❖ Bring the oven to 375 heat setting.
- ❖ Cut the squash, lengthwise, into 4 steaks.
- ❖ Carefully core one side of each squash with a paring knife in a crosshatch
- ❖ Pattern.
- ❖ Use a brush, coat with olive oil each side of the steak
- ❖ Then season generously with salt and pepper.
- ❖ In an oven-safe, non-stick skillet, bring 2 tablespoons of olive oil to a warm temperature.
- ❖ Place the steaks on the skillet with the cored side down
- ❖ Cook at medium temperature until browned, approximately 5 minutes.
- ❖ Flip and repeat on the other side for about 3 minutes.
- ❖ Place the skillet into the oven to roast the squash for 7 minutes.

- ❖ Take out from the oven, placing on a plate
- ❖ Cover with aluminum foil to keep warm.
- ❖ Use the previously used skillet, add thyme, garlic, and shallot, cooking at medium heat
- ❖ Stir frequently for about 2 minutes.
- ❖ Add brandy and cook for an additional minute.
- ❖ Next, add paprika and whisk the mixture together for 3 minutes
- ❖ Then in the yogurt seasoning with salt and pepper.
- ❖ Plate the steaks and spoon the sauce over the top.
- ❖ Garnish with parsley and enjoy!

64) CAULIFLOWER STEAK KICKING CORN

Preparation Time: 30 min   **Cooking Time:** 60 min.   **Servings: 6**

Ingredients:
- ✓ 2 t. Capers, drained
- ✓ 4 scallions, chopped
- ✓ 1 red chili, minced
- ✓ ¼ c. Vegetable oil

Ingredients:
- ✓ 2 ears of corn, shucked
- ✓ 2 big cauliflower heads
- ✓ Salt and pepper to taste

Directions:
- ❖ Heat the oven to 375 degrees.
- ❖ Boil a pot of water, about 4 cups, using the maximum heat setting available
- ❖ Add corn in the saucepan, cooking approximately 3 minutes or until tender
- ❖ Drain and allow the corn to cool, then slice the kernels away from the cob
- ❖ Warm 2 tablespoons of vegetable oil in a skillet.
- ❖ Combine the chili pepper with the oil, cooking for approximately 30 seconds
- ❖ Next, combine the scallions, sautéing with the chili pepper until soft.
- ❖ Mix in the corn and capers in the skillet

- ❖ Warm 1 tablespoon of vegetable oil in a skillet
- ❖ Once warm, begin to place cauliflower steaks to the pan, 2 to 3 at a time
- ❖ Season to your liking with salt
- ❖ Cook over medium heat for 3 minutes or until lightly browned.
- ❖ Once cooked, slide onto the cookie sheet
- ❖ Take the corn mixture and press into the spaces between the florets of the cauliflower.
- ❖ Bake for 25 minutes. Serve warm and enjoy!
- ❖ Cook for approximately 1 minute to blend the flavors. Then remove from heat.

65) PISTACHIO WATERMELON STEAK

Preparation Time: 5 min   **Cooking Time:** 10 min.   **Servings: 4**

Ingredients:
- ✓ Microgreens pistachios chopped
- ✓ Malden sea salt
- ✓ 1 tbsp. Olive oil, extra virgin

Ingredients:
- ✓ 1 watermelon
- ✓ Salt to taste

Directions:
- ❖ Begin by cutting the ends of the watermelon.
- ❖ Carefully peel the skin from the watermelon along the white outer edge
- ❖ Slice the watermelon into 4 slices, approximately 2 inches thick.
- ❖ Trim the slices, so they are rectangular in shape approximately 2 x4 inches

- ❖ Heat a skillet to medium heat add 1 tablespoon of olive oil.
- ❖ Add watermelon steaks and cook until the edges begin to caramelize
- ❖ Plate and top with pistachios and microgreens.
- ❖ Sprinkle with malden salt. Serve warm and enjoy!

66) BBQ RIBS

Preparation Time: 30 min   **Cooking Time:** 45 min.   **Servings: 2**

Ingredients:
- ✓ 2 drops liquid smoke
- ✓ 2 tbsp. Of the following: soy sauce
- ✓ Tahini
- ✓ 1 c. Of the following: water
- ✓ Wheat gluten
- ✓ 1 tbsp. Of the following:
- ✓ Garlic powder onion powder lemon pepper
- ✓ 2 t. Chipotle powder
- ✓ For the sauce:
- ✓ 2 chipotle peppers in adobo, minced
- ✓ 1 tbsp. Of the following:
- ✓ Vegan worcestershire sauce lemon juice

Ingredients:
- ✓ Horseradish onion powder
- ✓ Garlic powder
- ✓ Ground pepper
- ✓ 1 t. Dry mustard
- ✓ 2 tbsp. Sweetener of your choice
- ✓ 5 tbsp. Brown sugar
- ✓ ½ c. Apple cider vinegar
- ✓ 2 c. Ketchup
- ✓ 1 c. Water
- ✓ 1 freshly squeezed orange juice

Directions:
- ❖ Set the oven to 350 heat setting, and prepare the grill charcoal as recommended for this, but gas will work as well.
- ❖ Combine soy sauce, tahini, water, and liquid smoke in a bowl
- ❖ Then set this mixture to the side in a mixing bowl.
- ❖ Next, use a big glass bowl to mix chipotle powder, onion powder
- ❖ Add lemon pepper, garlic powder; combine well
- ❖ Whisk in the ingredients from the little bowl.
- ❖ Add the wheat gluten and mix until it comes to a gooey consistency.
- ❖ Grease a standard-size loaf pan and transfer the mixture to the loaf pan
- ❖ Smooth it out so that the rib mixture fits flat in the pan.
- ❖ Bake for 30 minutes.

- ❖ While the mixture is baking, make the bbq sauce
- ❖ To make the sauce, combine all the sauce ingredients in a pot
- ❖ Allow the mixture to simmer its way to the boiling point to combine the flavors
- ❖ As soon as it boils, decrease the heat to the minimum setting
- ❖ Let it be for 10 more minutes.
- ❖ Cautiously take the rib out of the oven and slide onto a plate.
- ❖ Coat the top rib mixture with the bbq sauce and place on the grill.
- ❖ Coat the other side of the rib mixture with bbq sauce and grill for 6 minutes
- ❖ Flip and grill the other side for an additional 6 minutes.
- ❖ Serve warm and enjoy!

67) SPICY VEGGIE STEAKS WITH VEGGIES

Preparation Time: 30 min   **Cooking Time**: 45 mins.   **Servings**: 4

Ingredients:
- ✓ 1 ¾ c. Vital wheat gluten
- ✓ ½ c. Vegetable stock
- ✓ ¼ t. Liquid smoke
- ✓ 1 tbsp. Dijon mustard
- ✓ 1 t. Paprika
- ✓ ½ c. Tomato paste
- ✓ 2 tbsp. Soy sauce
- ✓ ½ t. Oregano
- ✓ ¼ t. Of the following:
- ✓ Coriander powder cumin
- ✓ 1 t. Of the following:
- ✓ Onion powder garlic powder
- ✓ ¼ c. Nutritional yeast

Ingredients:
- ✓ 2 cloves garlic, minced
- ✓ 2 tbsp. Soy sauce
- ✓ 1 tbsp. Lemon juice, freshly squeezed
- ✓ ¼ c. Maple syrup for skewers:
- ✓ 15 skewers, soaked in water for 30 minutes if wooden
- ✓ ¾ t. Salt
- ✓ 8 oz. Zucchini or yellow summer squash
- ✓ ¼ t. Ground black pepper
- ✓ 1 tbsp. Olive oil
- ✓ 1 red onion, medium
- ✓ ¾ c. Canned chickpeas marinade:
- ✓ ½ t. Red pepper flakes

Directions:
- ❖ In a food processor, add chickpeas, vegetable stock, liquid smoke, dijon mustard, pepper
- ❖ Then paprika, tomato paste, soy sauce, oregano, coriander, cumin, onion powder, garlic, and natural yeast
- ❖ Process until the ingredients are well- mixed.
- ❖ Add the vital wheat gluten to a big mixing bowl,
- ❖ Pour the contents from the food processor into the center
- ❖ Mix with a spoon until a soft dough is formed.
- ❖ Knead the dough for approximately 2 minutes; do not over knead.
- ❖ Once the dough is firm and stretchy, flatten it to create 4 equal-sized steaks.
- ❖ Individually wrap the steaks in tin foil;
- ❖ Be sure not to wrap the steaks too tightly, as they will expand when steaming.
- ❖ Steam for 20 minutes. To steam, use any steamer or a basket over boiling water.
- ❖ While steaming, prepare the marinade.

- ❖ In a bowl, whisk the red pepper, garlic, soy sauce, lemon juice, and syrup
- ❖ Reserve half of the sauce for brushing during grilling. Prepare the skewers.
- ❖ Cut the onion and zucchini or yellow squash into 1/2-inch chunks.
- ❖ In a glass bowl, add the red onion, zucchini, and yellow squash
- ❖ Then coat with olive oil, pepper, and salt to taste
- ❖ Place the vegetables on the skewers.
- ❖ After the steaks have steamed for 20 minutes, unwrap and place on a cookie sheet
- ❖ Pour the marinade over the steaks, fully covering them.
- ❖ Bring your skewers, steaks, and glaze to the grill
- ❖ Place the skewers on the grill over direct heat
- ❖ Brush skewers with glaze. Grill for approximately 3 minutes then flip.
- ❖ Place the steaks directly on the grill, glaze side down
- ❖ Brush the top with additional glaze, Cook to your desired doneness.
- ❖ Serve warm and enjoy!

68) TOFU FAJITA BOWL

Preparation Time: 5minutes   **Cooking Time:** 10minutes   **Servings: 4**

Ingredients:
- ✓ 2 tbsp olive oil
- ✓ 1½ lb tofu, cut into strips
- ✓ Salt and ground black pepper to taste
- ✓ 2 tbsp tex-mex seasoning
- ✓ 1 small iceberg lettuce, chopped
- ✓ 2 large tomatoes, deseeded and chopped

Directions:
- ❖ Heat the olive oil in a medium skillet over medium heat
- ❖ Season the tofu with salt, black pepper, and tex-mex seasoning
- ❖ Fry in the oil on both sides until golden and cooked, 5 to 10 minutes. Transfer to a plate.

Ingredients:
- ✓ 2 avocados, halved, pitted, and chopped
- ✓ 1 green bell pepper, deseeded and thinly sliced
- ✓ 1 yellow onion, thinly sliced
- ✓ 4 tbsp fresh cilantro leaves
- ✓ ½ cup shredded dairy- free parmesan cheese blend
- ✓ 1 cup plain unsweetened yogurt
- ❖ Divide the lettuce into 4 serving bowls, share the tofu on top
- ❖ Add the tomatoes, avocados, bell pepper, onion, cilantro, and cheese.
- ❖ Top with dollops of plain yogurt and serve immediately with low carb tortillas.

69) INDIAN STYLE TEMPEH BAKE

Preparation Time: 10minutes   **Cooking Time:** 26minutes   **Servings: 4**

Ingredients:
- ✓ 3 tbsp unsalted butter
- ✓ 6 tempeh, cut into
- ✓ 1-inch cubes
- ✓ Salt and ground black pepper to taste

Directions:
- ❖ Preheat the oven to 350 f and grease a baking dish with cooking spray. Set aside.
- ❖ Heat the ghee in a medium skillet over medium heat
- ❖ Season the tempeh with salt and black pepper
- ❖ Cook in the oil on both sides until golden on the outside, 6 minutes.

Ingredients:
- ✓ 2 ½ tbsp garam masala
- ✓ 1 cup baby spinach, tightly pressed
- ✓ 1¼ cups coconut cream
- ✓ 1 tbsp fresh cilantro, finely chopped
- ❖ Add the spinach, and spread the coconut cream on top.
- ❖ Bake in the oven for 20 minutes or until the cream is bubbly.
- ❖ Remove the dish, garnish with cilantro
- ❖ Serve with cauliflower couscous.
- ❖ Mix in half of the garam masala and transfer the tempeh (with juicesinto the baking dish.

70) TOFU- SEITAN CASSEROLE

Preparation Time: 10minutes   **Cooking Time:** 20minutes   **Servings: 4**

Ingredients:
- ✓ 1 tofu, shredded
- ✓ 7 oz seitan, chopped
- ✓ 8 oz dairy- free cream cheese (vegan 1 tbsp dijon mustard

Directions:
- ❖ Preheat the oven to 350 f and grease a baking dish with cooking spray. Set aside.
- ❖ Spread the tofu and seitan in the bottom of the dish.
- ❖ In a small bowl, mix the cashew cream, dijon mustard
- ❖ Add vinegar, and two- thirds of the cheddar cheese

Ingredients:
- ✓ 1 tbsp plain vinegar
- ✓ 10 oz shredded cheddar cheese
- ✓ Salt and ground black pepper to taste
- ❖ Spread the mixture on top of the tofu and seitan
- ❖ Season with salt and black pepper, and cover with the remaining cheese.
- ❖ Bake in the oven for 15 to 20 minutes or until the cheese melts and is golden brown.
- ❖ Remove the dish and serve with steamed collards

71) SAGE QUINOA

Preparation Time: 10 minutes   **Cooking Time**: 30 minutes   **Servings: 4**

Ingredients:
- ✓ 1 tablespoon olive oil
- ✓ 1 yellow onion, chopped
- ✓ 1 cup quinoa
- ✓ 2 cups chicken stock

Directions:
- ❖ Heat up a pan with the oil over medium-high heat
- ❖ Add the onion and the garlic and sauté for 5 minutes.

Ingredients:
- ✓ 1 tablespoon sage, chopped
- ✓ 2 garlic cloves, minced
- ✓ A pinch of salt and black pepper
- ✓ 1 tablespoon chives, chopped
- ❖ Then the quinoa and the other ingredients, toss
- ❖ Cook over medium heat for 25 minutes more
- ❖ Divide between plates and serve.

72) BEANS, CARROTS AND SPINACH SIDE DISH

Preparation Time: 10 minutes   **Cooking Time**: 4 hours   **Servings: 6**

Ingredients:
- ✓ 5 carrots, sliced
- ✓ 1 and ½ cups great northern beans, dried, soaked overnight and drained
- ✓ 2 garlic cloves, minced
- ✓ 1 yellow onion, chopped
- ✓ Salt and black pepper to the taste
- ✓ ½ teaspoon oregano, dried

Directions:
- ❖ In your slow cooker, mix beans with onion, carrots, garlic, salt
- ❖ Then pepper, oregano and veggie stock
- ❖ Stir, cover and cook on High for 4 hours.
- ❖ Drain beans mix, return to your slow cooker
- ❖ Reserve ¼ cup cooking liquid.
- ❖ Add spinach, lemon juice and lemon peel

Ingredients:
- ✓ 5 ounces baby spinach
- ✓ 4 and ½ cups veggie stock
- ✓ 2 teaspoons lemon peel, grated 3 tablespoons lemon juice
- ✓ 1 avocado, pitted, peeled and chopped
- ✓ ¾ cup tofu, firm, pressed, drained and crumbled
- ✓ ¼ cup pistachios, chopped
- ❖ Stir and leave aside for 5 minutes.
- ❖ Transfer beans, carrots and spinach mixture to a bowl
- ❖ Then pistachios, avocado, tofu
- ❖ Reserve cooking liquid, toss
- ❖ Divide between plates and serve. Enjoy!

73) SCALLOPED POTATOES

Preparation Time: 10 minutes   **Cooking Time**: 4 hours   **Servings: 8**

Ingredients:
- ✓ Cooking spray
- ✓ 2 pounds gold potatoes, halved and sliced
- ✓ 1 yellow onion, cut into medium wedges
- ✓ 10 ounces canned vegan potato cream soup
- ✓ 8 ounces coconut milk

Directions:
- ❖ Coat your slow cooker with cooking spray
- ❖ Arrange half of the potatoes on the bottom.
- ❖ Layer onion wedges, half of the vegan cream soup, coconut milk
- ❖ Add tofu, stock, salt and pepper.
- ❖ Then the rest of the potatoes, onion wedges

Ingredients:
- ✓ 1 cup tofu, crumbled
- ✓ ½ cup veggie stock
- ✓ Salt and black pepper to the taste
- ✓ 1 tablespoons parsley, chopped

- ❖ Join also cream, coconut milk, tofu and stock,
- ❖ Cover and cook on High for 4 hours.
- ❖ Sprinkle parsley on top
- ❖ Divide scalloped potatoes between plates
- ❖ Serve and enjoy!

74) SWEET POTATOES SIDE DISH

Preparation Time: 10 minutes   **Cooking Time**: 3 hours   **Servings: 10**

Ingredients:
- ✓ 4 pounds sweet potatoes, thinly sliced
- ✓ 3 tablespoons stevia
- ✓ ½ cup orange juice
- ✓ A pinch of salt and black pepper

Directions:
- ❖ Arrange potato slices on the bottom of your slow cooker.
- ❖ In a bowl, mix orange juice with salt, pepper, stevia
- ❖ Then thyme, sage and oil and whisk well.

Ingredients:
- ✓ ½ teaspoon thyme, dried
- ✓ ½ teaspoon sage, dried
- ✓ 2 tablespoons olive oil

- ❖ Add this over potatoes, cover slow cooker
- ❖ Cook on High for 3 hours.
- ❖ Divide between plates. Serve!

75) CAULIFLOWER AND BROCCOLI SIDE DISH

Preparation Time: 10 minutes   **Cooking Time:** 3 hours   **Servings: 10**

Ingredients:
- ✓ 4 cups broccoli florets
- ✓ 4 cups cauliflower florets
- ✓ 14 ounces tomato paste
- ✓ 1 yellow onion, chopped

Directions:
- ❖ In your slow cooker, mix broccoli with cauliflower, tomato paste
- ❖ Then onion, thyme, salt and pepper

Ingredients:
- ✓ 1 teaspoon thyme, dried
- ✓ Salt and black pepper to the taste
- ✓ ½ cup almonds, sliced

- ❖ Toss, cover and cook on High for 3 hours.
- ❖ Add almonds, toss, divide between plates. Serve.

76) WILD RICE MIX

Preparation Time: 10 minutes   **Cooking Time:** 6 hours   **Servings: 12**

Ingredients:
- ✓ 40 ounces veggie stock
- ✓ 2 and ½ cups wild rice
- ✓ 1 cup carrot, shredded
- ✓ 4 ounces mushrooms, sliced
- ✓ 2 tablespoons olive oil

Directions:
- ❖ In your slow cooker, mix stock with wild rice, carrot, mushrooms
- ❖ Add oil, marjoram, salt, pepper, cherries, pecans and green onions

Ingredients:
- ✓ 2 teaspoons marjoram, dried and crushed
- ✓ Salt and black pepper to the taste
- ✓ 2/3 cup dried cherries
- ✓ ½ cup pecans, toasted and chopped
- ✓ 2/3 cup green onions, chopped

- ❖ Toss, cover and cook on Low for 6 hours.
- ❖ Stir wild rice one more time, divide between plates
- ❖ Serve and enjoy!

77) RUSTIC MASHED POTATOES

Preparation Time: 10 minutes   **Cooking Time**: 4 hours   **Servings: 6**

Ingredients:
- ✓ 6 garlic cloves, peeled
- ✓ 3 pounds gold potatoes, peeled and cubed
- ✓ 1 bay leaf
- ✓ 1 cup coconut milk

Directions:
- ❖ In your slow cooker, mix potatoes with stock, bay leaf
- ❖ Then garlic, salt and pepper
- ❖ Cover and cook on High for 4 hours.

Ingredients:
- ✓ 28 ounces veggie stock
- ✓ 3 tablespoons olive oil
- ✓ Salt and black pepper to the taste

- ❖ Drain potatoes and garlic, return them to your slow cooker
- ❖ ash using a potato masher.
- ❖ Add oil and coconut milk, whisk well
- ❖ Divide between plates. Serve!

78) GLAZED CARROTS

Preparation Time: 10 minutes   **Cooking Time**: 4 hours   **Servings: 10**

Ingredients:
- ✓ 1 pound parsnips, cut into medium chunks
- ✓ 2 pounds carrots, cut into medium chunks
- ✓ 2 tablespoons orange peel, shredded
- ✓ 1 cup orange juice
- ✓ ½ cup orange marmalade

Directions:
- ❖ In your slow cooker, mix parsnips with carrots.
- ❖ In a bowl, mix orange peel with orange juice
- ❖ Then stock, orange marmalade
- ❖ Add tapioca, salt and pepper

Ingredients:
- ✓ ½ cup veggie stock
- ✓ 1 tablespoon tapioca, crushed
- ✓ A pinch of salt and black pepper
- ✓ 3 tablespoons olive oil
- ✓ ¼ cup parsley, chopped

- ❖ Whisk and add over carrots.
- ❖ Cover slow cooker and cook everything on High for 4 hours.
- ❖ Then parsley, toss
- ❖ Divide between plates. Serve

79) MUSHROOM AND PEAS RISOTTO

Preparation Time: 10 minutes   **Cooking Time**: 1 hour and 30 minutes   **Servings: 8**

Ingredients:
- ✓ 1 shallot, chopped
- ✓ 8 ounces white mushrooms, sliced
- ✓ 3 tablespoons olive oil
- ✓ 1 teaspoon garlic, minced

Directions:
- ❖ In your slow cooker, mix oil with shallot, mushrooms, garlic
- ❖ Add rice, stock, peas, salt and pepper

Ingredients:
- ✓ 1 and ¾ cup white rice
- ✓ 4 cups veggie stock
- ✓ 1 cup peas
- ✓ Salt and black pepper to the taste
- ❖ Stir, cover and cook on High for 1 hour and 30 minutes.
- ❖ Stir risotto one more time
- ❖ Divide between plates. Serve!

80) SQUASH AND SPINACH MIX

Preparation Time: 10 minutes

Cooking Time: 3 hours and 30 minutes

Servings: 12

Ingredients:
- ✓ 10 ounces spinach, torn
- ✓ 2 pounds butternut squash, peeled and cubed
- ✓ 1 cup barley
- ✓ 1 yellow onion, chopped

Directions:
- ❖ In your slow cooker, mix squash with spinach, barley, onion
- ❖ Add stock, water, salt, pepper and garlic

Ingredients:
- ✓ 14 ounces veggie stock
- ✓ ½ cup water
- ✓ A pinch of salt and black pepper to the taste
- ✓ 3 garlic cloves, minced

- ❖ Toss, cover and cook on High for 3 hours and 30 minutes.
- ❖ Divide squash mix on plates
- ❖ Serve and enjoy!

DESSERT RECIPES

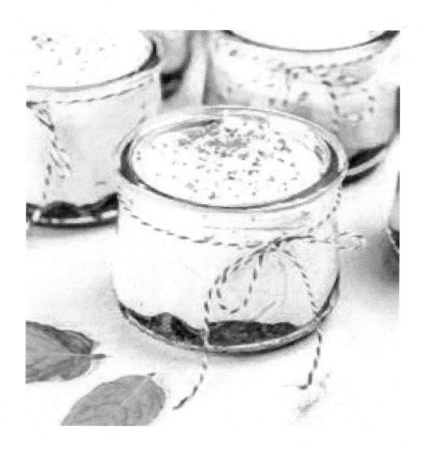

81) DATES MOUSSE

Preparation Time: 30 minutes   **Cooking Time:** 0 minutes   **Servings: 4**

Ingredients:
- ✓ 2 cups coconut cream
- ✓ ¼ cup stevia
- ✓ 2 cups dates, chopped

Ingredients:
- ✓ 1 teaspoon almond extract
- ✓ 1 teaspoon vanilla extract

Directions:
- ❖ In a blender, combine ingredients
- ❖ Pulse well, minutes before serving.

- ❖ Add the cream with the stevia, dates and the other ingredientes
- ❖ Divide into cups and keep in the fridge for 30

82) MINTY ALMOND CUPS

Preparation Time: 10 minutes   **Cooking Time:** 10 minutes   **Servings: 4**

Ingredients:
- ✓ 1 cup almonds, roughly chopped
- ✓ 1 tablespoon mint, chopped
- ✓ ½ cup coconut cream

Ingredients:
- ✓ 2 tablespoons stevia
- ✓ 1 teaspoon vanilla extract

Directions:
- ❖ In a pan, combine the almonds with the mint, the cream
- ❖ Add the other ingredients

- ❖ Whisk, simmer over medium heat for 10 minutes
- ❖ Divide into cups and serve cold.

83) LIME CAKE

Preparation Time: 10 minutes   **Cooking Time:** 40 minutes   **Servings: 4**

Ingredients:
- ✓ ½ cup almonds, chopped
- ✓ Zest of 1 lime grated
- ✓ Juice of 1 lime
- ✓ 1 cups stevia
- ✓ 2 tablespoons flaxseed mixed with

Ingredients:
- ✓ 3 tablespoons water
- ✓ 1 teaspoon vanilla extract
- ✓ 1 and ½ cup almond flour
- ✓ ½ cup coconut cream
- ✓ 1 teaspoon baking soda

Directions:
- ❖ In a bowl, combine the almond with the lime zest, lime juice
- ❖ Add the other ingredients
- ❖ Whisk well and pour into a cake pan lined with parchment paper.

- ❖ Introduce in the oven at 360 degrees F
- ❖ Bake for 40 minutes, cool down, slice and serve.

84) VANILLA PUDDING

Preparation Time: 10 minutes   **Cooking Time:** 40 minutes   **Servings: 4**

Ingredients:
- ✓ 2 cups almond flour
- ✓ 3 tablespoons walnuts, chopped
- ✓ 1 and ½ cups coconut cream
- ✓ 3 tablespoons flaxseed mixed with 4 tablespoons water

Ingredients:
- ✓ 1 cup stevia
- ✓ 1 teaspoon vanilla extract
- ✓ 1 teaspoon baking powder
- ✓ 1 teaspoon nutmeg, ground

Directions:
- ❖ In a bowl, combine the flour with the walnuts, the cream
- ❖ Add the other ingredients
- ❖ Whisk well and pour into 4 ramekins.

- ❖ Introduce in the oven at 350 degrees F
- ❖ Bake for 40 minutes, cool down and serve.

85) CINNAMON AVOCADO AND BERRIES MIX

Preparation Time: 5 minutes   **Cooking Time**: 0 minutes   **Servings: 4**

Ingredients:
- ✓ 1 cup blackberries
- ✓ 1 cup strawberries, halved
- ✓ 1 cup avocado, peeled, pitted and cubed

Directions:
- ❖ In a bowl, combine the berries with the avocado
- ❖ Add the other ingredients

Ingredients:
- ✓ 1 cup coconut cream
- ✓ 1 teaspoon cinnamon powder
- ✓ 4 tablespoons stevia

- ❖ Toss, divide into smaller bowls and serve cold.

86) RAISINS AND BERRIES CREAM

Preparation Time: 5 minutes   **Cooking Time:**   **Servings: 4**

Ingredients:
- ✓ 1 cup coconut cream
- ✓ 1 cup blackberries
- ✓ 3 tablespoons stevia

Directions:
- ❖ In a blender, the cream with the berries and the other ingredients except the raisins

Ingredients:
- ✓ 2 tablespoons raisins
- ✓ 2 tablespoons lime juice

- ❖ Pulse well, divide into cups, sprinkle the raisins on top and cool down before serving.

87) BAKED RHUBARB

Preparation Time: 10 minutes   **Cooking Time:** 20 minutes   **Servings: 4**

Ingredients:
- ✓ 4 teaspoons stevia
- ✓ 1 pound rhubarb, roughly sliced
- ✓ 1 teaspoon vanilla extract

Directions:
- ❖ Arrange the rhubarb on a baking sheet lined with parchment paper
- ❖ Add the stevia, vanilla and the other Ingredients

Ingredients:
- ✓ 2 tablespoons avocado oil
- ✓ 1 teaspoon cinnamon powder
- ✓ 1 teaspoon nutmeg, ground

- ❖ Toss and bake at 350 degrees F for 20 minutes.
- ❖ Divide the baked rhubarb into bowls and serve cold.
- ❖ Nutrition: calories 176, fat 4.5, fiber 7.6, carbs 11.5, protein 5

88) COCOA BERRIES MOUSSE

Preparation Time: 10 minutes   **Cooking Time:** 0 minutes   **Servings: 2**

Ingredients:
- ✓ 1 tablespoon cocoa powder
- ✓ 1 cup blackberries
- ✓ 1 cup blueberries

Directions:
- ❖ In a blender, combine the berries with the cocoa and the other ingredients

Ingredients:
- ✓ ¾ cup coconut cream
- ✓ 1 tablespoon stevia

- ❖ Pulse well, divide into bowls and keep in the fridge for 2 hours before serving.

89) NUTMEG PUDDING

Preparation Time: 10 minutes   **Cooking Time:** 20 minutes   **Servings: 6**

Ingredients:
- ✓ 2 tablespoons stevia
- ✓ 1 teaspoon nutmeg, ground
- ✓ 1 cup cauliflower rice

Ingredients:
- ✓ 2 tablespoons flaxseed mixed with 3 tablespoons water
- ✓ 2 cups almond milk
- ✓ ¼ teaspoon nutmeg, grated

Directions:
- ❖ In a pan, combine the cauliflower rice with the flaxseed mix
- ❖ Add the other ingredients

- ❖ Whisk, cook over medium heat for 20 minutes
- ❖ Divide into bowls and serve cold.

90) LIME CHERRIES AND RICE PUDDING

Preparation Time: 10 minutes   **Cooking Time:** 25 minutes   **Servings: 4**

Ingredients:
- ✓ ¾ cup stevia
- ✓ 2 cups coconut milk
- ✓ 3 tablespoons flaxseed mixed with
- ✓ 4 tablespoons water Juice of 2 limes

Ingredients:
- ✓ Zest of 1 lime, grated
- ✓ 1 cup cherries, pitted and halved
- ✓ 1 cup cauliflower rice

Directions:
- ❖ In a pan, combine the milk with the stevia
- ❖ Bring to a simmer over medium heat.
- ❖ Add the cauliflower rice and the other ingredients

- ❖ Stir, cook for 25 minutes more
- ❖ Divide into cups and serve cold.

91) ALMOND BALLS

Preparation Time: 10 minutes   **Cooking Time:** 0 minutes   **Servings: 6**

Ingredients:
- ✓ ½ cup coconut oil, melted
- ✓ 5 tablespoons almonds, chopped

Ingredients:
- ✓ 1 tablespoon stevia
- ✓ ¼ cup coconut flesh, unsweetened and shredded

Directions:
- ❖ In a bowl, combine the coconut oil with the almonds
- ❖ Add the other Ingredients

- ❖ Stir well and spoon into round moulds.
- ❖ Serve them cold.

92) GRAPEFRUIT CREAM

Preparation Time: 10 minutes   **Cooking Time:** 0 minutes   **Servings: 4**

Ingredients:
- ✓ 2 cups coconut cream
- ✓ 1 cup grapefruit, peeled, and chopped

Ingredients:
- ✓ 2 tablespoons stevia
- ✓ 1 teaspoon vanilla extract

Directions:
- ❖ In a blender, combine the coconut cream with the grapefruit

- ❖ Add the other ingredients
- ❖ Pulse well, divide into bowls and serve cold.

93) TANGERINE STEW

Preparation Time: 10 minutes   **Cooking Time:** 10 minutes   **Servings: 4**

Ingredients:
- ✓ 1 cup coconut water
- ✓ 2 cups tangerines, peeled and cut into segments
- ✓ 1 tablespoon lime juice

Ingredients:
- ✓ 1 tablespoon stevia
- ✓ ½ teaspoon vanilla extract

Directions:
- ❖ In a pan, combine the coconut water with the tangerines
- ❖ Add the other ingredients

- ❖ Toss, bring to a simmer and cook over medium heat for 10 minutes.
- ❖ Divide into bowls and serve cold.

94) WATERMELON MOUSSE

Preparation Time: 10 minutes   **Cooking Time:** 0 minutes   **Servings: 4**

Ingredients:
- ✓ 1 cup coconut cream
- ✓ 1 tablespoon lemon juice

Ingredients:
- ✓ 1 tablespoon stevia
- ✓ 2 cups watermelon, peeled and cubed

Directions:
- ❖ In a blender, combine the watermelon with the cream

- ❖ Add the lemon juice and stevia
- ❖ Pulse well, divide into bowls and serve cold.

95) FRUIT SALAD

Preparation Time: 2 hours   **Cooking Time:** 0 minutes   **Servings: 4**

Ingredients:
- ✓ 2 avocados, peeled, pitted and cubed
- ✓ ½ cup blackberries
- ✓ ½ cup strawberries, halved
- ✓ ½ cup pineapple, peeled and cubed

Ingredients:
- ✓ ¼ teaspoon vanilla extract
- ✓ 2 tablespoons stevia
- ✓ Juice of 1 lime

Directions:
- ❖ In a bowl, combine the avocados with the berries

- ❖ Add the other ingredients
- ❖ Toss and keep in the fridge for 2 hours before serving.

96) CHIA BARS

Preparation Time: 10 minutes   **Cooking Time:** 20 minutes   **Servings: 6**

Ingredients:
- ✓ 1 cup coconut oil, melted
- ✓ ½ teaspoon baking soda
- ✓ 3 tablespoons chia seeds
- ✓ 2 tablespoons stevia

Ingredients:
- ✓ 1 cup coconut cream
- ✓ 3 tablespoons flaxseed mixed with
- ✓ 4 tablespoons water

Directions:
- ❖ In a bowl, combine the coconut oil with the cream
- ❖ Add the chia seeds and the other ingredients
- ❖ Whisk well, pour everything into a square baking dish

- ❖ Introduce in the oven at 370 degrees F and bake for 20 minutes.
- ❖ Cool down, slice into squares and serve.

97) FRUITS STEW

Preparation Time: 10 minutes　　　**Cooking Time:** 10 minutes　　　**Servings: 4**

Ingredients:
- ✓ 1 avocado, peeled, pitted and sliced
- ✓ 1 cup plums, stoned and halved
- ✓ 2 cups water

Directions:
- ❖ In a pan, combine the avocado with the plums, water
- ❖ Add the other ingredients

Ingredients:
- ✓ 2 teaspoons vanilla extract
- ✓ 1 tablespoon lemon juice
- ✓ 2 tablespoons stevia

- ❖ Bring to a simmer and cook over medium heat for 10 minutes.
- ❖ Divide the mix into bowls and serve cold.

98) AVOCADO AND RHUBARB SALAD

Preparation Time: 10 minutes　　　**Cooking Time:** 0 minutes　　　**Servings: 4**

Ingredients:
- ✓ 1 tablespoon stevia
- ✓ 1 cup rhubarb, sliced and boiled
- ✓ 2 avocados, peeled, pitted and sliced

Directions:
- ❖ In a bowl, combine the rhubarb with the avocado

Ingredients:
- ✓ 1 teaspoon vanilla extract
- ✓ Juice of 1 lime

- ❖ Add the other ingredients, toss and serve.

99) PLUMS AND NUTS BOWLS

Preparation Time: 5 minutes　　　**Cooking Time:** 0 minutes　　　**Servings: 2**

Ingredients:
- ✓ 2 tablespoons stevia
- ✓ 1 cup walnuts, chopped

Directions:
- ❖ In a bowl, mix the plums with the walnuts

Ingredients:
- ✓ 1 cup plums, pitted and halved
- ✓ 1 teaspoon vanilla extract

- ❖ Add the other ingredients
- ❖ Toss, divide into 2 bowls and serve cold.

100) AVOCADO AND STRAWBERRIES SALAD

Preparation Time: 5 minutes　　　**Cooking Time:** 0 minutes　　　**Servings: 4**

Ingredients:
- ✓ 2 avocados, pitted, peeled and cubed
- ✓ 1 cup strawberries, halved
- ✓ Juice of 1 lime

Directions:
- ❖ In a bowl, combine the avocados with the strawberries

Ingredients:
- ✓ 1 teaspoon almond extract
- ✓ 2 tablespoons almonds, chopped
- ✓ 1 tablespoon stevia

- ❖ Add the other Ingredients, toss and serve.

Thanks for reading this book

CPSIA information can be obtained
at www.ICGtesting.com
Printed in the USA
BVHW010653180621
609821BV00015B/239